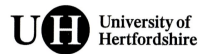

University of Hertfordshire

College Lane, Hatfield, Herts. AL¹

Learning and Informati⌐ ⌐

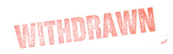

A Casebook of Cognitive Behaviour Therapy for Command Hallucinations

Command hallucinations are a particularly distressing and sometimes dangerous type of hallucination about which relatively little is known and for which no evidence-based treatment currently exists.

In *A Casebook of Cognitive Behaviour Therapy for Command Hallucinations* the development of a new and innovative evidence-based cognitive therapy is presented in a practical format ideal for the busy practitioner. This new approach is based on over a decade's research on the role of voice hearers' beliefs about the power and omnipotence of their voices and how this drives distress and 'acting on' voices. The therapy protocol is presented in clear steps from formulation to intervention. The body of the book describes its application in eight cases illustrating the breadth of its application, including 'complex' cases. The authors also present their interpretation of what their findings tell us about what works and doesn't work, and suggestions for future developments. Subjects covered also include:

- Understanding command hallucinations.
- A cognitive versus a quasi-neuroleptic approach to CBT in psychosis.
- Does CBT for CH work? Findings from a randomised controlled trial.

This book provides a fascinating and very practical summary of the first intervention to have a major impact on distress and on compliance with command hallucinations. It will be of great interest to all mental health practitioners working with people with psychosis in community and forensic settings.

Sarah Byrne is a clinical psychologist working in adult mental health services in Warwickshire.

Max Birchwood is Professor of Mental Health at the University of Birmingham and Director of the Birmingham Early Intervention Service.

Peter E. Trower is Honorary Associate Professor in the School of Psychology, University of Birmingham and Consultant Clinical Psychologist for Birmingham and Solihull Mental Health Trust.

Alan Meaden is a consultant specialist clinical psychologist in Rehabilitation and Continuing Needs for Birmingham and Solihull Mental Health Trust.

A Casebook of Cognitive Behaviour Therapy for Command Hallucinations

A social rank theory approach

Sarah Byrne, Max Birchwood, Peter E. Trower and Alan Meaden

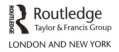

LONDON AND NEW YORK

First published 2006
by Routledge
27 Church Road, Hove, East Sussex BN3 2FA

Simultaneously published in the USA and Canada
by Routledge
270 Madison Ave, New York, NY 10016

Routledge is an imprint of the Taylor & Francis Group

Typeset in Times by RefineCatch Ltd, Bungay, Suffolk
Printed and bound in Great Britain by Biddles Ltd, King's Lynn
Cover design by Sandra Heath

This publication has been produced with paper manufactured to
strict environmental standards and with pulp derived from
sustainable forests.

British Library Cataloguing in Publication Data
A catalogue record for this book is available from the British Library

Library of Congress Cataloging-in-Publication Data
A casebook of cognitive behaviour therapy for command
hallucinations : a social rank theory approach / Sarah Byrne . . . [et al.].
    p. ; cm.
  Includes bibliographical references and index.
  ISBN 1-58391-785-3 (hbk)
  1. Auditory hallucinations–Treatment. 2. Schizophrenia–
Treatment. 3. Cognitive therapy. 4. Auditory hallucination–
Treatment–Case studies. 5. Schizophrenia–Treatment–
Case studies. 6. Cognitive therapy–Case studies.
  [DNLM: 1. Hallucinations–therapy–Case Reports. 2. Cognitive
Therapy–methods–Case Reports. 3. Dominance-Subordination–
Case Reports. 4. Models, Psychological–Case Reports. 5.
Schizophrenia–therapy–Case Reports. WM 204 C337 2006]
I. Byrne, Sarah. II. Title.

RC553.A84C37 2006
616.89'142–dc22

               2005015699

ISBN10: 1-58391-785-3

ISBN13: 9-78-1-58391-785-3

Contents

List of authors   vii
Preface   ix
Acknowledgements   xi

1 Understanding command hallucinations   1

2 A cognitive versus a quasi-neuroleptic approach   10

3 Cognitive behaviour therapy for command hallucinations:
  a manual   14

4 Tom   31

5 Joan   39

6 Tony   50

7 Naomi   60

8 Janice   70

9 Sally   89

10 Kevin   99

11 Does CBT for CH work? Findings from a randomised
   controlled trial   111

Epilogue   120

References 121
Appendices 125
Index 139

Authors

Sarah Byrne is a practising clinical psychologist, working in adult mental health in Stratford-upon-Avon. Prior to this, she was an Honorary Research Associate in the School of Psychology at the University of Birmingham, working on the randomised controlled trial of cognitive therapy for command hallucinations. She was the sole therapist in the trial, as well as being involved in the development and writing of the therapy protocol, in developing appropriate measures and in day-to-day monitoring of progress. As a result of this research, she is co-author of two papers and one book chapter.

Max Birchwood is Professor of Mental Health at the University of Birmingham and Director of the Birmingham Early Intervention service. Together with colleagues he has undertaken pioneering work in cognitive behaviour therapy (CBT) for psychosis, including: the cognitive model of voices; cognitive therapy in acute psychosis and for command hallucinations; the prediction and control of relapse using 'early signs'; and the concept of the relapse signature. His current interests involve developing the concept and practice of early intervention and in understanding the developmental pathways to emotional dysfunction in psychosis.

Peter Trower is Honorary Associate Professor in the School of Psychology, University of Birmingham and Consultant Clinical Psychologist for Birmingham and Solihull Mental Health Trust. He is an Associate Fellow and accredited supervisor in rational emotive behaviour therapy. He has carried out research over a 30-year period including social skills training, social anxiety disorder and CBT for psychosis, and has over 80 publications.

Alan Meaden is a consultant specialist clinical psychologist in Rehabilitation and Continuing Needs for Birmingham and Solihull Mental Health Trust. He takes a lead role in promoting psychological approaches to working with individuals affected by psychosis in rehabilitation and assertive outreach services. He has carried out research into service issues and psychological approaches to understanding and treating psychosis over the past 10 years. His current interests include supportive psychotherapy and working with staff groups, and, of course, CBT.

Preface

Thirty-three-year-old Ralph heard three male voices every day. No one was actually there. They were all hallucinations. But Ralph believed they were very real, and very distressing. They always said things that were extremely critical and alarming, including personal threats to himself (e.g. 'we are going to stab you') and personal verbal abuse ('you are a pervert'; 'you are evil'). Most seriously of all they commanded Ralph to do terrible things to himself and others, to harm or kill. For example, they would say 'kill yourself, you deserve to die'; 'go and get a hammer'; 'kill X (someone who abused him when he was young)'; 'kill your Dad'. Not surprisingly, Ralph felt extremely frightened. He heard the voices at least once a day, particularly at night, often lasting for hours at a time. He felt that he had no choice but to listen to them. As we shall see, he sometimes felt compelled to obey some of them, and sometimes to resist but to appease them when he did so. At other times he coped by shouting and swearing at the voices, listening to the TV or radio and drinking alcohol.

This book is about command hallucinations of the type that Ralph experienced. As our brief description shows, command hallucinations are particularly distressing and potentially dangerous. As a proportion of hallucinations that many people with a diagnosis of schizophrenia have, they are surprisingly common, as we shall show. Yet relatively little is known about them compared to other symptoms of severe mental illness. What we do know is not encouraging, particularly that they are often intractable and resistant to traditional forms of treatment, and as a consequence people with command hallucinations may have to be compulsorily detained in hospital and retained, for example, in semi-secure forensic units in order to protect them and others from harm.

It became clear to many clinicians in the field that a better understanding of command hallucinations and an effective form of intervention based on such a model was sorely needed. Equally pressing was the need, once such an approach was developed, to make it widely available to clinicians who work with clients who suffer from command hallucinations.

Over a number of years a team of us at the University of Birmingham,

England, have worked on developing a theoretical model of command hallucinations with direct relevance to the development of a new form of cognitive behavioural intervention based on this model. After initial promising results with Ralph and a few other single cases, we undertook a platform trial, which encouragingly confirmed our initial findings. We intend to evaluate this therapy further in a full-scale multi-centre randomised controlled trial, but believe that in the meantime we have sufficiently good results to feel the time is right to make our treatment method available. And that is mainly what this book is about – it's a practice manual for troublesome and distressing command hallucinations.

In the book we describe this new and innovative cognitive therapy in detail, including the rationale and theory that informed the therapy, assessment (including a battery of assessment instruments, many of which were devised for this population), formulation and intervention. We then describe the application of the intervention in eight cases, chosen for their variability in order to illustrate the adaptations required to modify the intervention for each case.

Finally, we describe the trial we conducted to evaluate the effectiveness of the intervention, and give our interpretation of what the findings tell us about what works and doesn't work, and suggestions for future developments.

Sarah Byrne
Max Birchwood
Peter Trower
Alan Meaden
July 2005

Acknowledgements

We are indebted to many people who contributed in various ways to the development of our cognitive behaviour therapy for command hallucinations programme. In particular we thank Professor Paul Gilbert from Derby University and Professor Paul Chadwick from Southampton Mental Health NHS Trust and the University of Southampton for their distinguished intellectual and model-building contributions, and Angela Nelson for her vital work on the trial. We also thank the clients who participated in our trial and the relatives and clinical staff who helped and supported us. Finally, thanks to our friends and colleagues on the command hallucinations 'torch' project at La Trobe University, Melbourne, Australia, for an invaluable exchange of ideas.

Chapter 1

Understanding command hallucinations

In schizophrenia research, considerable progress has been made in recent years towards understanding the psychological and interpersonal characteristics of hallucinations. In this context, one particular class of hallucinations, namely command hallucinations (CHs) has recently become a focus of theory, research and clinical intervention. Indeed, the importance of CHs has become clear for both theoretical reasons – the light that these symptoms throw on the psychological nature of positive symptoms in general – and practice reasons, since CHs are one of the most high-risk and distressing, but intractable and drug-resistant, symptoms of schizophrenia.

What are command hallucinations? CHs have long been recognised but little understood, with few effective interventions. The key feature that distinguishes them from ordinary hallucinations is that phenomenologically the voice is experienced or interpreted as commanding rather than commenting. The perceived commands range from making a harmless gesture to behaving in ways that are potentially injurious or lethal to self or others. Although there is general agreement on these features in the literature (indeed Bleuler (1924:62) referred to command hallucinations having a 'compulsive power' making them difficult to ignore), very little in the way of specific diagnostic guidelines is available, and they are not specifically mentioned in DSMIV (American Psychiatric Association, 1994). There is clearly a need for such guidelines, for example whether the term CHs should be confined to voices where there is an explicit command or whether it should include voices where the client *interprets* that a command is implied. In our approach we have adopted the latter criterion. As we shall describe later, we have also developed our own rating for severity of command, and a risk assessment grading system for degree of compliance or resistance.

How common are CHs in general? In a recent review, Shawyer *et al.* (2003) found eight studies reporting the prevalence of CHs in samples of adult psychiatric patients with auditory hallucinations. The median prevalence rate for these studies is 53 per cent, but with a very wide range of 18 to 89 per cent. Equivalent prevalence rates in forensic populations were no higher.

How common are dangerous or harmful CHs? Shawyer *et al.* (2003) report a median prevalence of 48 per cent for harmful CHs in non-forensic patients with CHs, i.e. roughly half, but again the range was considerable, from 7 to 70 per cent. Forensic groups were almost certainly much higher, with 83 per cent of voice hearers found to have CHs with 'criminal' content.

How common is compliance with dangerous or harmful CHs? This is the question of most concern to clinicians. A median prevalence of at least partial compliance to harmful CHs is 31 per cent in community samples, though yet again the range is very wide (0–92 per cent (Shawyer *et al.*, 2003)) and therefore the picture is far from clear. In the forensic population results suggested that rates were higher. In summarising, Shawyer *et al.* said the evidence suggests that CHs may be associated in a complex manner with violence. Nonetheless, harmful CHs to hurt others and to hurt self have been found to be associated with an increased risk of violence toward others and self-harm respectively.

The figures quoted above clearly show that patients don't always comply with their commanding voices, and we know from our own research that they sometimes refuse altogether and sometimes resist but comply in a symbolic or minor way as a gesture of appeasement to the voice. Why they respond in these varying ways is a vitally important issue that we explore in detail later. At this point we simply want to illustrate the kinds of commands that are heard and the range of responses elicited. We obtained an indication of these data from our recent trial (see Chapter 11) in which all 38 patients who entered the trial reported two or more commands – at least one of which was a 'severe' command – and had recently complied with the command. The most severe commands were to kill self (25), kill others (13), harm self (12) and harm others (14). Less severe commands involved innocuous, day-to-day behaviour (wash dishes, masturbate, take a bath) and minor social transgressions (break windows, shout out loud, swear in public). Further details including incidence and examples of compliance and appeasement of these commands for the sample as a whole are shown in Table 1.1.

What kind of therapy is provided and what is effective? It won't come as a surprise that this patient group requires and, on the whole, receives a major and inevitably expensive share of mental health service resources. Apart from specialist services such as forensic services and detention in semi-secure units, this group receives input from virtually every relevant professional and type of service, both inpatient and outpatient. We found, for example, that no fewer than 19 categories of service were provided for the 38 patients in our trial, reported in Chapter 10. So provision is expensive, but is it effective? There is little definitive data on this question, and what there is is not encouraging. Sawyer *et al.* found that patients who complied with their CHs were receiving significantly higher doses of antipsychotic medication than those who did not comply, suggesting that medication may have been ineffective in suppressing their CHs. Indications are that CHs feature strongly in those considered 'treatment resistant' and even hospitalisation is not necessarily a barrier to

Table 1.1 Prevalence of and types of commands, compliance and appeasement in a sample of 38 individuals with command hallucinations[1]

Command and prevalence	Example	Compliance	Appeasement
Command to kill self (n = 25)	'stab yourself' 'slash your wrists' 'overdose' 'hang yourself' 'gas yourself'	Nine patients had previously attempted suicide. One patient committed suicide during the trial.	Seven patients used appeasement behaviours including holding a knife to their wrist, taking razor blades into the bath, collecting tablets and planning and executing suicide in their imagination.
Command to kill others (n = 13)	'cut her throat' 'go and kill someone' 'kill the therapist' 'kill your husband and daughter'	Four patients in the sample had attempted to kill someone, by suffocation, poisoning or physical assault with a hammer.	Three patients used appeasement behaviours including arming themselves with knives, baseball bats and an axe and making guns out of tin foil.
Command to harm self (n = 12)	'burn yourself' 'cut yourself' 'set yourself alight' 'pour hot water on yourself' 'go into the road'	Nine patients had harmed themselves in response to commands. This included cutting, swallowing nail polish remover or bleach, jumping in front of cars, walking on glass and setting oneself alight.	Three patients used appeasement behaviours including picking at previous wounds, and standing on the kerb.
Command to harm others (n = 14)	'touch your children' 'kick them' 'hit them' 'beat that person up' 'rape your neighbour'	Seven patients had harmed others in response to commands. This included hitting children, knocking them into furniture, scolding them, hitting people, attacking someone with a knife.	Two patients used appeasement behaviours including hitting others with minimal force, and covert appeasement by thinking 'I'll do that later'.

[1] Reproduced with permission of the Royal College of Psychiatrists. Originally published in Trower, P. et al. (2004). Cognitive therapy for command hallucinations. *British Journal of Psychiatry*, 184, 312–320.

compliance (e.g. Jones *et al.*, 1992). Hospitalisation obviously reduces risk to the public but it simply restricts physical opportunities to act on CHs and can hardly be considered an effective 'therapy' for the individual. In our trial (Trower *et al.*, 2004) we report the very high medication dose that is commonly used, its propensity to creep upwards over time and the absence of a link between drug dose and compliance behaviour. So, in summary, services are expensive but probably not very effective.

The link between CHs and harm to self or others is not straightforward, however. Population studies suggest that people with a diagnosis of schizophrenia are more at risk of harm to self and to others (Brennan *et al.*, 2000) than those without psychosis, but the link between the *form* of individual symptoms and the risk of individuals *acting* on these has proved difficult to establish (Milton *et al.*, 2001; Appelbaum *et al.*, 2000; Buchanan, 1993), including the risk associated with the presence of command hallucinations in the MacArthur study (Appelbaum *et al.*, 2000). Some argue that there is no link between the presence of command hallucinations and 'dangerous behaviour' (Rudnick-Abraham, 1999); but the MacArthur study is not without its critics (Maden, 2003). However, we have argued (Braham *et al.*, 2004) that these population studies focus on the form of the command hallucination and ignore the content and the nature of the individual's *relationship* with his voice, which we discuss later.

A cognitive model for CHs

It is often assumed that symptoms such as hallucinations and associated affect and behaviour such as compliance are directly causally related within the syndrome of schizophrenia. However, as we have already seen, there is considerable variation in CHs between the command and the emotional and behavioural response to the command, such that there has to be some mediating variable between the two. In a critical review of the literature, Braham *et al.* (2004) found that the relationship between command and compliance was mediated by a number of factors, including beliefs about the voice's identity, familiarity, power and intent. The studies reviewed support the view that the beliefs that an individual holds about their voice will influence compliance, and that a cognitive model is required to explain the relationships and guide clinical intervention. In a cognitive model of hallucinations, Chadwick and Birchwood (1994) and Birchwood and Chadwick (1997) showed empirically that the distressing affect and behaviour arising from hallucinations may be understood as a function not simply of the content or topography of voice activity but also of voice hearers' appraisal of their meaning. One of the key insights in this model, drawn and adapted from rational emotive behaviour therapy, is to view the hallucination as an activating event (A), whose significance is appraised by the individual in terms of their belief system (B), and which largely gives rise to characteristic emotional and behaviour

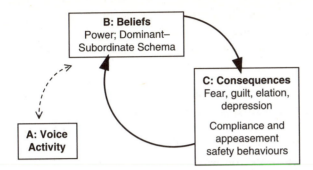

Figure 1.1 Command hallucinations–compliance cycle. Flow diagram illustrating the effect of power beliefs (B) on distress and compliance (C) when triggered by voice activity (A), in a continuous, self-maintaining cycle. Based on social rank theory (Gilbert, 1992) and a cognitive model of voices (Chadwick and Birchwood, 1994).

consequences (C). This is illustrated in Figure 1.1. Here we show voice activity as the activating event that triggers the key beliefs of power and dominance/subordination (explained below). These beliefs give rise, according to our cognitive theory, to the consequences – principally the emotions of fear, guilt and depression and sometimes elation, and the behaviours of compliance or appeasement. These behaviours can be construed as 'safety' behaviours – part of a cognitive mechanism that maintains the belief in the power of the voice, which we explain below. Chadwick and Birchwood (1994) found evidence for this type of cognitive mediation in the maintenance of beliefs about voices: in many cases, belief content was 'at odds' with voice content, suggesting that meanings are constructed by individuals rather than directly voice-driven. Indeed, participants in this study disclosed what was for them compelling evidence for their beliefs, which only occasionally drew upon voice content. These results were replicated by Van der Gaag *et al.* (2003).

A second discovery from this body of research has, we believe, thrown radically new light on the nature of the appraisal of voices. This is the finding that the distress and behaviour linked to voice activity may be understood in terms of the nature of patients' perceived relationship with their voices, in particular their personification of them and their appraisal of voices' 'power and omnipotence' and whether the voice is malevolent or benevolent (Chadwick and Birchwood, 1994). The key variables in this relationship can be summarised under the headings of power, identity and meaning. Power refers to beliefs the individual makes about how much they can or cannot control the voice and how much they believe they need to comply (see Figure 1.1). Identity refers to beliefs about 'who' the voice is: often this is a supernatural force, the Devil or God or a spirit. Meaning refers to beliefs about the voice's intent – that the voice must be obeyed or it will punish the person.

Recent research has found empirical support for the centrality of the power differential between voice and voice hearer in the level of distress and also coping strategies (Birchwood *et al.*, 2000). This model has explanatory value when one considers the risk of compliance with command hallucinations. Junginger (1990) found that recent compliance was more likely where the individual personified, or attributed an identity to, the voice. Over 85 per cent of voice hearers see the voice as powerful and omnipotent whereas, by contrast, the hearer is usually perceived as weak and dependent, unable to control or influence the voice (Birchwood and Chadwick, 1997). Thus, it was found that the greater the perceived power and omnipotence of the voice, the greater the likelihood of compliance (Beck-Sander *et al.*, 1997). This relationship is not linear and was moderated by appraisal of the consequences of resisting the voice on one hand, and the consequences of social transgression on the other. Results showed that those with benevolent voices virtually always complied with the voice, irrespective of whether the command was socially 'innocuous' or 'severe' (Beck-Sander *et al.*, 1997). Furthermore, we have argued that the relationship with the voice is a paradigm or mirror of social relationships in general, such that individuals who feel subordinate to the powerful voice also feel subordinate to others in their social world (Birchwood *et al.*, 2000, 2004).

From these and other studies we can now assert with some confidence the following findings.

1   Voice hearers construct the link between themselves and their voice as having the nature of an intimate interpersonal relationship and often one that is inescapable (Benjamin, 1989). In a cross-sectional study, Junginger (1990) found that recent compliance was more likely where the individual personified the voice (i.e. attributed it to an identity).

2   More than 85 per cent of voice hearers see the voice as powerful and omnipotent, whereas the hearer is usually weak and dependent, unable to control or influence the voice (Birchwood and Chadwick, 1997). This is particularly the case among those seen in psychiatric services.

3   More than two-thirds of voice hearers were at least moderately depressed, which was directly attributable to the interpersonal appraisal of power and entrapment by the voice (Birchwood and Chadwick, 1997) and to social appraisals of powerlessness and low social status (Birchwood *et al.*, 2004).

4   The greater the perceived power and omnipotence of the voice compared to the voice hearer, the greater was the likelihood of compliance (Beck-Sander *et al.*, 1997), though this relationship is not linear and is moderated by appraisal of the voice's intent and consequences of resisting.

5   Voice hearers perceive the voice as omniscient (e.g. as knowing the person's present thoughts and past history, able to predict the future), and this was seen as proof of the voice's power.

6   Some voice hearers construed their voice as benevolent; others as malevolent and persecutory.(Chadwick and Birchwood, 1994; Birchwood and Chadwick, 1997).

7   Those with benevolent voices virtually always complied with the voice, irrespective of whether the command was 'innocuous' or 'severe' (Beck-Sander *et al.*, 1997), whereas those with malevolent voices were more likely to resist, and this resistance increased if the command involved major social transgression or self-harm (Birchwood and Chadwick, 1997). However, subjects predicted that the malevolent voice would inflict harm whenever they resisted, and, if they continued to resist, felt compelled to appease the voice by carrying out an alternative action.

8   The individuals engaged in behaviour viewed as likely to appease the powerful voice (e.g. compliance in imagination, or expressing *intent* to comply); these appeasements act as safety behaviours to (a) reduce the threat posed by the voice and (b) prevent disconfirmation of the belief. This is illustrated in Figure 1.1. We call these behaviours 'safety behaviours' because the voice hearer regards them as 'saving' him from the dominant voice's wrath, and the punishment he would otherwise experience. This cycle ensures that the client's belief in the power of the voice is never disconfirmed (indeed, it tends to be reinforced).

The cognitive model of voices enabled us to realise that it was the appraisal of voices rather than the voices *per se* that gave rise to distress and disturbed behaviour; the model also enabled the discovery through research that the key beliefs concerned power, obedience, identity and meaning. However, the model didn't explain *why* voice hearers had those particular beliefs. For example, it didn't explain why Ralph – introduced in the preface to this book and described in detail in Chapter 3 – had specific beliefs to obey the commands, let alone related beliefs such as resistance and appeasement. In other words, it didn't explain the content of the beliefs, and for a case conceptualisation that would help us to develop an assessment, formulation and intervention protocol – our goal – we needed such an explanation.

One of the insights noted earlier that helped towards this explanation was that our clients had a *relationship* with their voice. They personified the voice, and interacted with it much like they would with significant others in their lives. It is the nature of this relationship that can be understood in terms of a theory from evolutionary psychology called social rank theory. This theory has already been developed to explain features of depression (e.g. Gilbert, 1992; Brown *et al.*, 1995), social anxiety (Trower and Gilbert, 1989) and post-psychotic depression (Rooke and Birchwood, 1998). In a nutshell, the theory states that we humans, and many group-living animals, have evolved a way of living in social groups with social ranks, and have inherited mental mechanisms for bringing this about. In all social ranks you have leaders and followers, but in some, which have been termed 'agonic', you have an extremely punitive social environment in which the leaders are hostile dominants who oppress their subordinates (followers) by the exercise of power and control and the threat of punishment. This theory proposes that individuals in such subordinate positions, when threatened by those more dominant, have evolved ways of coping with and de-escalating threat, including a variety of interpersonal behaviours loosely labelled as appeasement and submission. These normally have the effect of terminating the aggression of the dominant and stabilising the relative rank differentials. Other subordinate characteristics include selective sensitivity to the commands of the dominant, a compulsion to obey such commands, and a compulsion to appease the dominants when obeying is risky or dangerous but escape is impossible. According to Paul Gilbert (1989), these social ranks are represented in the mind as dominant–subordinate cognitive schemas (see Figure 1.1) or what he calls mentalities, and some vulnerable individuals will perceive most social relationships in these terms.

When we come to formulate Ralph's problem in social rank theory terms we find that it fits uncannily well, in that Ralph perceives the voice as the dominant and himself as the subordinate. On a version of the Social Comparison Scale – a scale commonly used to measure the perceived social rank differential, that is how much one sees the other as up-rank and oneself as down-rank – we found that he rated the voice right at the top and himself at the bottom on such attributes as power, strength, respect, knowledge, superiority and ability to inflict harm. He believed that the voices were very powerful because he had no control over them; they were frequent, loud and persistent; if they told him something, it must be true, and they had taken over his mind. Furthermore he had taken two overdoses in response to the voices, and had cut his wrists superficially in order to appease the voices. He reported feeling compelled to obey the voices but had resisted commands to kill others for fear of being put in prison, although he feared that he would act on the commands if they continued to be so distressing.

However, we still have the question of how Ralph developed this schema, if we are not to assume that it is simply a symptom of the illness. Social rank theory helps here too, because the theory states that early developmental experiences of 'agonic' dominant–subordinate relationships will sensitise the individual to tend to interpret certain future relationships in those terms. This gives a specific content to Beck's point that dysfunctional schemas lie dormant until activated by current events that bear similarities to the original. So, one prediction of social rank theory is that a person who has, for example, been victimised early in life by an abusive dominant will carry that 'agonic' dominant–subordinate social rank perspective into adulthood as a dysfunctional schema. This is almost certainly what happened to Ralph, who was sexually abused at the age of nine; then, presumably, when he was put in a new agonic environment with his youth custody sentence, the schema was activated. By itself it doesn't account for the emergence of the voice, but it does account for the relationship with the voice, and with significant others in his environment. It can be construed as a cognitive vulnerability – a dominant–subordinate schema – imprinted during early learning, being triggered by a current incident and leading to the perception of the dominant other, subordinate self, triggered currently by a relationship with the voice and significant others who in some way resemble the earlier persecutor. Then, more specifically in Ralph's case, we have the early dominant abuser and himself the subordinate victim, currently triggered by the voice which is perceived as equivalent to the persecutor (Ralph said that one of the voices was that of the abuser). One of the beliefs is 'I must comply or be punished', giving rise to extreme anxiety and compliance, or resistance with appeasement behaviour. This cycles back, of course, reinforcing the perception of the powerful voice since he is preventing himself from discovering that actually the voice can do nothing.

In two large-scale studies, we have shown that the relationship with the voice is a paradigm or mirror of social relationships in general, such that individuals who feel subordinate to the powerful voice also feel subordinate to others in their social world (Birchwood *et al.*, 2000, 2004). In other words, the perceived dominant–subordinate relationship between voice and voice hearer may be driven by individuals' core interpersonal schema.

In this framework, the key independent variable is the perceived power – indeed omnipotence – of the personified voice: the greater the perceived power differential between voice and voice hearer, the greater is the probability of complying with the 'benevolent' voices, and of complying with, or resisting and appeasing, 'malevolent' voices, depending on the nature (severity) of the command. Thus, the cognitive model of CHs proposes that high-risk behaviours of people with CHs are a consequence of beliefs, namely a conviction in the power of their voices, a belief that they are compelled to comply with and appease these voices, a belief that to resist will lead to worse consequences for self or others; and that these beliefs are underpinned by core interpersonal schemas of inferiority.

In summary, we have presented in this opening chapter our cognitive behaviour therapy (CBT) for CH model of CHs, which combines the cognitive model of hallucinations and social rank theory. The model has, we believe, important implications for guiding the way we develop and practice cognitive therapy, and this approach differs from much of that in the literature on CBT for psychosis. This is the topic of our next chapter, and prepares the ground for the subsequent chapters on therapy and research.

Chapter 2

A cognitive versus a quasi-neuroleptic approach

The rapidity with which CBT has become an established therapy for schizophrenia is remarkable. Some 15 years ago CBT was widely regarded as quite inappropriate for this, the severest mental illness, and was nowhere available as far as we know. Then a few pioneering research groups, mainly in the UK and Australia, re-ignited the very early work that Beck (1952) and others had done in the 1950s but that had remained dormant for decades. Some exciting and unexpected results came from this work. For example, Chadwick and Lowe (1990) surprised many with their finding, using multiple baseline single-case methodology, that it was possible to engage people with psychosis in a collaborative fashion and to explore systematically the logical and empirical bases for their delusions. This process of 'collaborative empiricism' was found to weaken strongly held delusional beliefs. The rest, as they say, is history. This and parallel work inspired clinical researchers to develop and implement CBT protocols for various aspects of psychosis, and this has led in turn to a proliferation of randomised controlled trials and an assured place for CBT in the therapeutic armamentarium (Pilling *et al.*, 2002; Tarrier and Wykes, 2004).

Taking its place in the context of this creative output is of course cognitive behaviour therapy for command hallucinations (CBT for CH) – one of the latest such developments, and the focus of this book. Despite early scepticism that CBT could make an impact on one of the most intractable problems in psychosis (i.e. CHs), we have found, in a randomised controlled trial (Trower *et al.*, 2004; Chapter 11, this volume) that it is indeed effective in reducing compliance and distress when undertaken according to our protocol (Byrne *et al.*, 2003; Chapter 3, this volume).

However, there is an important difference in the direction we have taken in developing CBT for CH from that reported in much of the outcome literature on CBT for psychosis. For although the modestly positive findings of that research have been encouraging, they may have been limited by what we argue is a questionable therapeutic goal and an equally questionable research strategy. In this chapter we outline our understanding of that goal and that research strategy, then we clarify what our recommended goal and strategy are. Finally, we compare the two and explain why we think that ours is the better strategy, both theoretically and clinically. The subsequent chapters can then hopefully be seen to follow and to illustrate our proposed strategy.

The majority of CBT for psychosis trials have as their goal the eradication or amelioration of the symptoms of psychosis. This is modelled on drug trials, which traditionally are aimed at reducing symptoms, and CBT based on this model can fairly be described as a 'quasi-neuroleptic', i.e. treating CBT as a kind of proxy drug that is also aimed at symptoms and that can be conveniently compared to medication, to see which is more effective. In this model the primary dependent variable (i.e. the variable the treatment is primarily aimed at changing) is the symptoms, as measured by traditional symptom rating scales, and the *secondary* dependent variables are the patients' distress (depression, anxiety) and dysfunctional behaviour. Distress and behaviour are secondary because they are deemed to be caused by the symptoms (or the illness) and, if the symptom is removed/reduced, they should be reduced.

Our recommended model is a truly cognitive as opposed to a quasi-neuroleptic model. As described in Chapter 1, the goal is not the eradication of symptoms *per se*, but the eradication or reduction of distress and dysfunctional behaviour. After all, from the patient's (and anyone else's) point of view, the symptoms only become important if they 'cause' distress for the patient or others (e.g. depression, anxiety) and dysfunctional behaviour (e.g. suicide, acting on dangerous commands). However, in a cognitive model it isn't so much the symptoms in themselves that 'cause' the distress and behaviour, but the patient's appraisal of them ('it is the voice of the Devil, it is all-powerful'). This is the ABC model that we outlined in Chapter 1, where the distress and behaviour are the C (consequences), symptoms are the A (activating event) and beliefs the B that 'cause' the C, given the A. Therefore CBT isn't targeted primarily at the symptoms (A) but rather the beliefs (B). By specifying precisely the beliefs that give rise to the consequences, we can test our hypothesis with precision. In the quasi-neuroleptic model, we suggest that not only is the wrong goal targeted but also the wrong cause, and aiming at the symptoms or illness at A, it is difficult to see how precise hypotheses about causal psychological mechanisms can be made. Whereas the cognitive model predicts specific B–C relationships that guide cognitive intervention to the specific Bs, the quasi-neuroleptic model predicts general A–C relationships that guide intervention to the symptoms/syndrome (A), with a loss of precision and power.

What is the evidence that most CBT for psychosis outcome research is based on a quasi-neuroleptic model? This is reflected in meta-analyses (Cormac *et al.*, 2002; Pilling *et al.*, 2002) where the Cochrane plots parallel those for studies of neuroleptics; indeed, the CBT trials reports are almost identical to pharmacological studies. CBT, in other words, is practised and evaluated within such trials as a quasi-neuroleptic with the same goal as neuroleptics of symptom reduction or removal. Studies have now appeared combining neu-roleptics and CBT on the assumption that they possess some functional equivalence (e.g. McGorry *et al.*, 2002). CBT for psychosis has nonetheless demonstrated efficacy in symptom reduction and led to the therapy being taken seriously by the mental health community and by research funders. However, effect sizes have been modest, particularly for distress and dys-functional behaviour where measured. We predict that a consequence of using our suggested cognitive model would be a considerable increase in the effect size for alleviation of distress and dysfunctional behaviour.

We looked at the 12 trials that had been published in peer-reviewed journals at the time of writing. The trials included were all those in the critical review by Pilling *et al.* (2002), plus four reported since 2002. These trials have shown a decisive impact on psychotic symptoms (Pilling *et al.*, 2002) with an effect size of 0.6 rising to 0.93 at follow-up (Gould *et al.*, 2001). Nine of the 12 trials measured depression as a secondary outcome. Four measured distress, using either the PSYRATS (Haddock *et al.*, 1999), which includes distress subscales, or the Personal Questionnaire Rating Scale Technique (PQRST: Brett-Jones *et al.*, 1987). In no study was distress separ-ately analysed (PSYRATS uses a distress scale to compile total scores for hallucinations or delusions).

Overall, three of the nine studies measuring depression reported an improvement in depression score attributed to CBT (Drury *et al.*, 1996; Sen-sky *et al.*, 2000; Turkington *et al.*, 2002). All of these were secondary meas-ures taken at the end of treatment, suggesting that the impact of the CBT on psychotic symptoms was responsible for a decrease in the depressed effect associated with them. Two studies described a longer-term improvement in depression at follow-up (Drury *et al.*, 1996; Sensky *et al.*, 2000). In the Drury *et al.* (1996) study, this may have reflected the attempt to challenge secondary appraisals of psychosis (e.g. loss, shame) that informed their CBT pro-gramme. Additionally, Tarrier *et al.* (2001) reported an improvement in mood following the alleviation of positive symptoms at the end of treatment. In summary, three out of the nine trials measuring depression reported that a reduction in the targeted psychotic symptoms was associated with a reduc-tion in depression (and in one case mood improvement: Tarrier *et al.*, 2001) at the end of therapy. The mean effect size of studies reporting a significant effect was 0.28, compared to the effect size of 0.65 (all studies) for psychotic symptoms (rising to 0.93 at follow-up) (Gould *et al.*, 2001). Of the four studies measuring delusional distress, one (Durham *et al.*, 2003) reported a reduction in the severity of delusions on the PSYRATS (the distress subscale is aggregated in the delusions scale score) and another (Kuipers *et al.*, 1998) reported an improvement in delusional distress (on PQRST) only at follow-up.

Considering the high level of depression and distress associated with posi-tive symptoms, and the scale of the impact of CBT on the positive symptoms, it is surprising that the impact of CBT on depression occurred in only a third of studies and with low effect size. These results call into question the assumption that easing distress and depression in psychosis will follow from the treatment of positive symptoms alone.

Returning to the opening theme of this chapter, we recommend a shift from a research strategy where CBT is treated as a quasi-neuroleptic to CBT as a truly *cognitive*-based therapy to relieve distress associated with psychotic experience and the 'co-morbid' emotional and behavioural dysfunctions. CBT has, we believe, a *distinctive* role to play in relieving distress, which is more in keeping with its natural roots in emotional dysfunction. This is what we have tried to do, both in our approach to therapy (Chapters 3 to 10) and in our trial (Chapter 11).

Cognitive behaviour therapy for command hallucinations

A manual

Following the principles of the cognitive model for voices and social rank theory described in Chapter 1, and our distinctive goals for research and practice outlined in Chapter 2, we developed cognitive behaviour therapy for command hallucinations (CBT for CH). We designed CBT for CH principally to enable clients to regain a sense of control over their actions by challenging the omnipotence of their voices, to reduce compliance by disconfirming the belief in severe consequences (e.g. belief that the voice will harm the client if they resist), and, most importantly, to ease distress associated with resistance. In this chapter we outline the CBT for CH procedure and illustrate it with a case study. We begin with the assessment stage.

Stage 1: The assessment stage

While the main purpose of this stage is assessment of psychotic symptoms, most notably CHs and their cognitive, behavioural and affective consequences, it includes a variety of tasks, namely engagement, assessment, formulation, promoting control and goal setting. Although the assessment stage is sequentially the first stage, the assessment process continues throughout therapy, and, as described below, forms part of an organic whole with intervention, since a major function of assessment is to evaluate the outcome of an intervention before further interventions are attempted. But we first have to be clear as to what we mean by 'commands'.

The definition of commands

Commands are defined as orders that the client experiences as emanating from a personified voice, which he believes he must obey. Some clients hear commands directly, such as 'set fire to the house', but, for others the command is interpreted indirectly from something the voice says, and the compulsion follows this interpretation. For example, one client hears a voice saying 'you smell'; she interprets this as meaning that she should shower/bathe immediately; for another client, when the voice says 'you will be on your way next week', he will pack a suitcase in preparation for the journey. Our definition of command, therefore, requires that the client interpret the voices as a command, not the clinical assessor nor the therapist.

Engagement

Engaging and retaining individuals in a therapeutic alliance is fundamental to any psychological therapy. However, engaging individuals who hear voices can be especially difficult due to the very distracting and distressing nature of CH experiences. Consequently there are particular as well as general principles that need to be deployed in the development of a sound therapeutic alliance. Key aspects of these sessions include:

- Establishing rapport and trust through empathic listening, being flexible about session arrangements (venues, times, shorter or longer sessions).
- Listening to and encouraging the client to give a detailed account of the experience of hearing voices and the beliefs the client has about his voices.
- Emphasising a commitment to the client and the client's priorities, especially helping the client to reduce the distress and disturbance she experiences due to hearing voices.
- Anticipating some of the problems concerning engagement and weakening and associated beliefs that could threaten the engagement process; for example, the client may be concerned about the expectations and pace of therapy or about being sectioned when disclosing information about symptoms.
- The use of a symbolic 'panic button' gives the client control over the process of therapy, with the option to disengage at any point.

The client may be unused to talking about her experiences and may feel anxious about doing so, for example thinking that the therapist will think it 'crazy' to have a commanding voice. The therapist needs to put the client at ease by giving explicit permission to talk openly about any issue.

The client may be reluctant to continue therapy due to his voices expressing anxiety about treatment or about the trustworthiness of the therapist. Anticipating that voices may comment adversely on the therapist will help the therapist develop strategies for keeping the client engaged.

Socialising the client into the 'cognitive' model

The idea of socialising the client into the cognitive model here is to begin the process of helping the client to distinguish between facts and beliefs, and to see that beliefs, unlike facts, can be true or false, and can be changed, especially when they are unhelpful. So, for example, it can be pointed out that it is a fact that the client has a commanding voice, but it is a belief of the client –

albeit strongly held – that the voice is omnipotent, or must be obeyed. The choice of example must be carefully considered. A good choice to start with would be a belief that the client has less than 100 per cent conviction in, and would be prepared to question. The value of this preparatory work at this early stage is to help the client gain some optimism for change and motivation to continue to work with the therapist.

Another strategy that can be introduced here is to develop a rationale for questioning voice beliefs by considering the advantages and disadvantages of the beliefs being true or false. Once the client sees that he would be 'better off' if the beliefs were false, his motivation to proceed with therapy will be increased.

Assessment and formulation

Assessment and formulation form the nub of stage 1, clearly preceding and giving direction to stage 2 intervention. However, in practice, assessment, formulation and intervention form a continuing reciprocal and iterative process. In these early sessions, the parameters of the belief system relating to the commanding voice are identified and formulated, but this will be modified in later sessions, and psychological origins and alternative formulations explored, as suggested below.

Four core beliefs define the client–voice power relationship and are explored in the early sessions. These are:

- *Power and control* (e.g. the belief that the voice is much more powerful than the voice hearer, and that the voice hearer does not have any control over the voice).
- *Compliance, resistance and appeasement* (e.g. the belief that the voice must be obeyed, and that, if resisted, the voice must be appeased, and that if neither obeyed nor sufficiently appeased, the voice can inflict harm on the voice hearer).
- *Voice identity* (e.g. the belief that the voice is God or the Devil).
- *Purpose and meaning* (e.g. the belief that the voice hearer is being punished by the voices for past behaviour).

The therapist uses these power belief concepts and the social rank theory framework to explore the client's beliefs about the voice. Assessment of these beliefs, and more general assessment of the client's symptoms and behaviours, are carried out mainly by interviewing the client in the manner described above, and by means of the following questionnaires and ratings, some of which have been specifically developed for this problem, and where indicated, are included in the appendices.

- *Beliefs about Voices Questionnaire* (BAVQ – Chadwick and Birchwood,

1995; BAVQ-R – Chadwick *et al.*, 2000). This measures key beliefs about auditory hallucinations including benevolence, malevolence and two dimensions of relationship with the voice: 'engagement' and 'resistance'. It, like its companion assessment *The Cognitive Assessment Schedule*, is usually completed on the most dominant voice: in this case, the most dominant commanding voice.

- *The Cognitive Assessment Schedule* (CAS – Chadwick and Birchwood, 1995) is used in conjunction with the BAVQ-R to assess further the individual's feelings and behaviour in relation to the voice, and his/her beliefs about the voice's identity, power, purpose or meaning and the likely consequences of obedience or resistance.

- *Voice Compliance Scale* (VCS – Beck-Sander *et al.*, Birchwood and Chadwick, 1997). This is an observer rated scale to measure specifically the frequency of CH and level of compliance/resistance with each identified command. This was developed as a research instrument, but for ordinary clinical assessment the clinician can obtain from the patient (or other informant, such as a relative) a description of all the commands and associated behaviours (compliance or resistance) within the previous eight weeks where they felt compelled to respond. The clinician then classifies each behaviour using the following scale: neither appeasement nor compliant (1); symbolic appeasement, i.e. compliant with innocuous and/or harmless commands (2); appeasement, i.e. preparatory acts or gestures (3); partial compliance with at least one severe command (4); full compliance with at least one severe command (5).

- *Voice Power Differential Scale* (VPDS – Birchwood *et al.*, 2000) (see Appendix 1). This measures the perceived relative power differential between the voice (usually the most dominant voice) and the voice hearer, with regard to the components of power including strength, confidence, respect, ability to inflict harm, superiority and knowledge. Each is rated on a five-point scale; they yield a total power score.

- *Omniscience Scale* (OS – Birchwood *et al.*, 2000). This scale measures the voice hearer's beliefs about her voices' knowledge regarding personal information.

In addition to these measures of the specific targeted beliefs for CH, we also routinely include more general measures for symptoms and distress including the following well-established scales.

- *Positive and Negative Syndrome Scale* (PANSS – Kay, Fiszbein and Opler, 1987). This is a widely used, well-established and comprehensive symptom-rating scale measuring mental state.

- *Psychotic Symptom Rating Scales* (PSYRATS – Haddock *et al.*, 1999) measure the severity of and distress associated with a number of dimensions of auditory hallucinations and delusions. The auditory hallucinations scales rate frequency, duration, location, loudness, beliefs re origin (external/internal), amount and degree of negative content, amount and intensity of distress, disruption to life and controllability. The delusions scales rate amount and duration of preoccupation, conviction, amount and intensity of distress and disruption to life. All scales are rated 0 (none) to 4 (extreme), and yield total scores for hallucinations and delusions.

- *Calgary Depression Scale for Schizophrenia* (CDSS – Addington *et al.*, 1993) is specifically designed for assessment of level of depression in people with a diagnosis of schizophrenia. It is a quick, reliable observer rating scale that does not overlap with negative symptoms, and measures depressed mood, hopelessness, self-depreciation, guilty ideas of reference, pathological guilt, morning depression, early wakening, elevated risk of attempted suicide and observed depression.
- *Risk of Acting on Commands Scale* (RACS, Appendix 2). This rating scale was specifically designed by the authors to identify the level of risk of acting on commands and the amount of distress associated with the commands, and to help monitor change in such levels as therapy progressed (see Appendix 2).

Administering these measures may form part of the engagement process itself, demonstrating an accurate attunement to the complexity of the client's difficulties and reinforcing the message that the client and her concerns are being taken seriously. The measures are most commonly conducted during the initial assessment phase and thus aid in the planning and initial targeting of interventions. We find repeating some measures more frequently helpful in gauging the impact of interventions (particularly those assessing affect, beliefs and behaviour), while more global measures of mental state and symptomatology may prove too intrusive to use repeatedly and may best be employed at the end of therapy and in any follow-up.

A further aid to evaluation of therapy has been developed as part of our randomised controlled trial of CBT for CH. The CBT for CH Therapy Adherence Protocol (see Appendix 3) enables an assessment to be made of the extent to which the therapist adheres to principles and practice of CBT for CH and offers a useful guide to the steps indicated for each stage of therapy. As such the protocol serves as a useful training aid and fidelity marker if used in conjunction with audio or video taping of therapy sessions.

Developing and sharing the formulation

The therapist's next task is to help the client to see that these power beliefs are the client's own beliefs about the voice. In this way the process of socialisation to the cognitive model, already started in the very first phase of engagement, is elaborated, and indeed continued throughout this assessment and throughout the whole process of therapy. The therapist makes a careful distinction (for herself and the client) between the voice as an activating event, e.g. what the voice actually says, and the client's interpretation of the voice content.

The therapist then develops a formulation around the theme of the identity and power differential between client and voice, with the consequent need to comply, or appease if resisted, and the fear of punishment if not obeyed or appeased. Having arrived at this formulation, the therapist's task is to propose it tentatively to the client (or preferably elicit it by Socratic questioning), with the aim of achieving a shared understanding.

If this shared understanding is achieved, therapist and client can then explore, perhaps at a later stage in therapy, the psychological origins of this power relationship, thus giving the client a convincing alternative formulation, which will further weaken the power of the voice. As this is as much an intervention as an assessment strategy, we describe its use later as part of stage 2. However, at this early stage the therapist may well be reformulating in her own mind, ready to use this strategy at the appropriate time. We can illustrate this point from one of our cases, David. The therapist hypothesised that David's beliefs about his voice arose from the trauma of a childhood rape. The beliefs were construed as reactions to, and attempts to make sense of, the hallucinatory experience. Associated evaluative themes related, on the one hand, to the client's sense of worthlessness and sense that he deserved punishment and, on the other, to anger at the abuser, whom he saw as abusing this trust. The therapist kept this tentative reformulation in the back of her mind ready to use as an intervention strategy when the time was right. Thus CBT for CH can be seen to involve a number of levels: initially working at the level of compliance, control and identity beliefs and later progressing to work on beliefs about meaning and purpose and their relationship to the person's beliefs about himself and others. Some clients may not reach this more advanced stage, and the therapist and client must make ongoing judgements about whether this stage of therapy is necessary or indeed desirable. The process of exploring and communicating the formulations – indeed the therapeutic process *per se* – involves utilising the skills of collaborative empiricism and guided discovery long established in cognitive therapy (e.g. Beck *et al.*, 1979), and didactic and Socratic techniques in rational emotive behaviour therapy (e.g. Dryden, 1995).

Promoting control

The process of promoting control involves developing or reinforcing a coping repertoire: by enhancing the person's existing coping strategies for reducing the distress associated with his voices, and introducing novel ideas that have been tried successfully by other voice hearers, such as learning to start and stop voices at will (see below). One useful strategy is to frame the voice and voice hearer as being in a relationship in which the client can develop boundaries. The aim is to help the client to have his own time (turn the voice off), to turn his attention to or away from the voice, and to make his own decisions, rather than always listening to and waiting for the voice to initiate decisions.

These coping strategies are used not only to bring some immediate relief and to help cement engagement, but also to start the process of gently challenging the power beliefs. Thus promoting control spans both stages – assessment and intervention – and underlines the fact that assessment and intervention are conceptually separate tasks but are clinically integrated activities.

Promoting control is designed to fulfil a number of aims:

- to emphasise the person's strengths in coping with their voices, and to start to build evidence against their powerlessness
- to highlight the person's ability to have some control over their voices, and thereby to build evidence against the voices' power
- to develop an understanding of factors that increase/decrease the presence of voices
- as a means of underpinning the therapeutic alliance.

Setting goals for therapy

The goals of therapy are to reduce the client's distress and compliance behaviour. The means to these goals is to identify and modify the power beliefs that, in a cognitive model, are largely responsible for the distress and behaviour. This involves identifying the client's current beliefs about her voices and developing a rationale to question them. These two tasks will usually have been facilitated in the steps outlined above. However, a key task in setting goals is to develop alternative beliefs and to use these to replace the existing ones. Table 3.1 gives examples of current and alternative beliefs in one case.

Table 3.1 Examples of current and alternative beliefs

Current beliefs	Alternative beliefs
• I must comply (at least partially) to prevent the voice harming me	• The voice cannot harm me, therefore I can choose to resist or ignore its commands
• I have no control over my voice	• I have learnt to have control over my voice by using the following coping strategies . . .
• My voice is powerful and therefore should be obeyed	• My voice is not powerful, so I do not have to obey it

By the end of stage 1, therefore, the client and therapist need to have a shared understanding of the following points.

Firstly, the goal is to reduce distress and compliance behaviour. This entails helping the client gain the insight that his distress and compliance are a consequence of his beliefs about the voices more than the voices *per se*. Therefore the client is encouraged to view the distress and behaviour as arising from beliefs about the voices, and not being an automatic product of the voice itself. The client is asked, for example, to imagine that his voice is an imposter and then asked whether he would feel/behave any differently if this were true.

Secondly, the beliefs can be changed, and the goal is to change them for functional alternatives. Beliefs about voices are not facts but hypotheses, i.e. inferences or interpretations that may or may not be true. The therapist draws on any doubts the client may have about her beliefs, or any changes in her interpretations over time, to help her see that her interpretations are neither definitive nor unchangeable. Alternative beliefs are developed, tested and adopted. The reason for questioning and testing beliefs in this way is to reduce distress and disturbance.

Stage 2: The intervention stage

The aim of this stage is to deconstruct explicitly the perceived power differential that we believe underpins the whole problem of compliance and distress that characterise command hallucinations. To be specific, the aim is to challenge the four power beliefs listed above, in order to:

- reduce the perceived power of the voice and increase the perceived power of the voice hearer
- reduce compliance and appeasement and increase resistance
- weaken the conviction about the identity of the voice
- weaken the conviction that the client is being, and will be, punished.

The general guideline is that the therapist does not challenge the client head-on but uses a variety of indirect tactics in the spirit of guided discovery. Having sown the seeds of belief questioning during the assessment phase, the therapist can hopefully now draw on the client's own doubt, past or present, the client's own contradictory evidence and behaviour, and the client's own concerns about the possibility that his beliefs about the voices may be wrong. The 'Columbo' technique is a particularly powerful form of Socratic questioning with an emphasis on curiosity, pointing out inconsistencies in a gentle, curious way (Fowler *et al.*, 1995).

Challenging the beliefs about voices

Challenging the dysfunctional beliefs includes questioning the client's evidence for the beliefs, following a line of logical reasoning that exposes inconsistencies in the client's beliefs, reality testing in a bid to disconfirm the beliefs, 'normalising' the voice qualities, and responding more assertively to the voice.

Questioning evidence

The routine procedure in cognitive therapy can be used here to list first evidence that supports, then evidence that goes against, the identified belief. Commonly the client will find it easier to provide supportive evidence, and help is often needed to build evidence against the belief. Such contradictory evidence can be built up from anything the client has noticed in the past that seemed to be inconsistent with what the voices said, including evidence that has been elicited during the course of therapy. The client is asked to rank-order evidence for and against each belief, from the most to least convincing. Evidence for the belief is questioned, starting with the least convincing evidence. The client is then asked to consider alternative explanations, and weigh the evidence for and against the alternatives. For example, one client, David, explored and was unable to find any evidence that the voice had ever harmed him, or, indeed, as a 'spirit', could possibly physically do so. He slowly came to realise that there was no basis for his belief that the voice could physically harm him and that he could therefore ignore its commands without fear of punishment.

Logical reasoning

This step involves developing a line of argument that moves in small steps, leading to the final step, which firmly challenges the belief. An important part of this exercise is to establish each of the key steps of the argument before they are connected together.

Reality testing of beliefs

Behavioural experiments can be used to test the validity of a belief. This entails carrying out or withholding a behaviour in order to test a prediction that something catastrophic will happen. This strategy is particularly useful, therefore, for testing beliefs that the voice will punish the client if she does not comply. For example, many clients develop appeasement strategies – that is, resisting more serious commands by enacting less serious behaviours. We view the use of appeasement as a safety behaviour preventing the individual from testing out the consequences of full non-compliance. The person is encouraged to reduce the degree of appeasement hand in hand with the promotion of her own power and control, and to discover that the feared outcome does not occur, hence weakening the belief. For example, having doubted his belief that the voice could harm him, David put this to the test by ignoring the commands, and, after several such tests, discovered that there were no consequences.

'Normalising' the voices

The client has personified and idealised the voice, resulting in beliefs around omnipotence and omniscience. Therapy aims to 'normalise' the voice, highlighting ways in which the voice is as fallible as any human being and therefore not, for example, God-like. Sometimes it may usefully be compared to nosy neighbours or school bullies, who crave attention and are best ignored.

Questioning the voice's command

Questioning the voice's command directly is an extension of the behavioural test. When the client is feeling more confident regarding his power-relationship with the voice, he may find it helpful to challenge the voice more assertively: for example, in response to a voice command, the client may ask 'Why should I do that? Why don't you do it yourself?' Such behavioural responses are designed to get the client to act against the dysfunctional power beliefs and in line with the new functional beliefs, thus further weakening the former and strengthening the latter.

Emphasising benefits of resistance

The therapist helps the client to identify the perceived consequences of carrying out a command compared with the perceived consequences of resisting it (e.g. short-term gains of reducing anxiety may be outweighed by long-term disadvantages). In pursuing this goal the therapist explores and challenges with the client the inferences that make the likelihood of severe punishment seem so compelling and certain. Where catastrophic beliefs are identified, for example, the therapist can explore the idea that obeying the command is a kind of safety behaviour preventing disconfirmation and these beliefs can be challenged and tested by the techniques described above.

Switching voices on and off

Once the person is able to take a more detached view of her subjective experience she can achieve a greater sense of control over the voices by learning to initiate and stop voice activity. This can be achieved using the following steps.

- Identify cues or strategies that increase and decrease the frequency and volume of voices.
- Practise the use of decreasing strategies within a session.
- Propose the notion that 'control' requires the demonstration that voice activity can be turned on as well as off; the analogy of learning to drive a car can be used, such that feeling in control of a car involves starting and stopping the car.
- The client is encouraged either to initiate or to increase voice activity for short periods, then reduce or stop it. These periods are then gradually lengthened. In the case of David, he learned to start and stop his voices at will. He could activate his voice within a session by reading a newspaper article referring to abuse (he had been abused as a child and the voice was activated by media references to child abuse). He was then able to stop the voice by talking about other matters.

Once the client has achieved some control, consider the implications for beliefs about the voices' omnipotence.

Increasing the perceived power of the voice hearer

Here the client identifies evidence of his own mastery and control. Most of the preceding interventions aimed at challenging the beliefs about the power of the voice will simultaneously and necessarily be proving that the client has mastery and control, not the voice. By Socratic questioning, the client can be made aware of this. For example the therapist can, by Socratic questioning, help the client discover he can ignore the voice's commands without punishment, can control the voice by switching the voice on and off and has the ability to care for himself and keep active in spite of the presence of distressing voices. The aim is to help the person to endorse his sense of mastery and control.

Reformulation

Sometimes it is possible to reformulate the explanation for the commanding voice not only in terms of the questionable power beliefs so far challenged, but also in terms of the psychological origins of the voice and even its identity, as we outlined in stage 1. This reformulation, skilfully handled and timed, can be a powerful *coup de grâce* with which to finally deconstruct the power and identity beliefs. In the case of David, having reached the stage of weakening the power beliefs by the methods so far described, the therapist explored the idea that the voice might not be Mr X speaking today, but a psychological reaction to the traumatic rape, a kind of reliving of the original experience. David slowly began to question his belief that the voice was Mr X, and to entertain the possibility that the voice was a response to difficult feelings triggered by specific events.

We now illustrate the steps of CBT for CH by describing how we used them to help Ralph. More detailed accounts, illustrating how CBT for CH can be adapted for different, and often difficult problems, are given in Chapters 4 to 9.

Ralph

Ralph is a 33-year-old man who began hearing voices at the age of 16. He reported being sexually abused at nine years of age. He was bullied by some of his peers, both physically and emotionally, and was tormented by them over the abuse. He became increasingly disruptive and difficult to manage, and was put into care at 14 years as his mother was unable to cope. At 16 he received a youth custody sentence for stealing; it was during this time that he began to hear voices. From 22 to 25 years of age he experienced remission from the voices but, since then, he has reported hearing them almost daily.

Stage 1: Assessment stage

During the initial assessment, Ralph reported hearing three male voices that were always distressing. The content of these voices was always unpleasant and negative, including personal threats to self (e.g. 'we are going to stab you'), personal verbal abuse relating to his self-concept (e.g. 'you are a pervert'; 'you are evil') and commands to self-harm and to harm others (e.g. 'kill yourself, you deserve to die'; 'go and get a hammer: kill X (Ralph's abuser)'; 'kill your Dad'). As a result, Ralph described feeling extremely frightened. Ralph said that he heard the voices at least once a day, particularly at night, often lasting for hours at a time. He felt that he had no choice but to listen to them. He coped by shouting and swearing at the voices, listening to the TV or radio and drinking alcohol.

The Voice Power Differential Scale (Birchwood *et al.*, 2000) showed that Ralph believed that the voices were much more powerful, stronger, more confident, more knowledgeable than him, superior to him, and much more capable of harming him than he was of defending himself. He believed that the voices were very powerful because:

- he had no perceived control over them
- of their frequency
- they said things in a loud, persistent way
- if they told him something, it must be true
- they had taken over his mind.

Beliefs about identity

Ralph reported being 100 per cent certain that one of the voices was that of his abuser, and that the other two were from the devil, because 'they sounded like them'.

Beliefs about purpose and meaning

Ralph believed that he was being persecuted by people for bad things in his past: he had committed burglary and theft as a young adult; he felt responsible for his mother's death; and he believed the voices were a punishment because he was sexually abused, for which, he believed, he bore responsibility.

Beliefs about compliance/resistance

Ralph had a past history of taking two overdoses in response to the voices, and he had previously cut his wrists superficially in order to appease the voices. He reported feeling compelled to obey the voices but had resisted commands to kill others for fear of being put in prison, although he feared acting on the commands if they continued to be so distressing. He acted on commands to get out of bed on the majority of occasions.

Beliefs about control

Ralph believed that he had some control over the voices, but only occasionally.

Target behaviours

The main compliance behaviour targeted for intervention was identified as 'acting on commands to harm himself or others', including wrist cutting (appeasement behaviour).

Stage 2: Intervention stage

Challenging beliefs about control over the voices

Supported by the therapist, Ralph developed a range of coping strategies that helped him to have more control over the voices: he found that talking to someone he trusted helped when the voices were distressing. Living in supported accommodation meant that he had access to support day and night if needed. Other helpful strategies included: telling the voices to stop or go away in a firm voice (out loud when alone, or to himself when in company); listening to the radio or watching football on TV; keeping active by meeting with friends; taking regular medication. These strategies were reinforced and it was suggested that these offered him some control.

Exploring the evidence for and against the power of the voices

Ralph began to believe that he had more control over the voices, using the above coping strategies. He used the evidence that he could cope as evidence to support an emerging belief that he had as much power as the voices.

Gradually, Ralph became aware that his voices often worsened (i.e. became louder, more frequent) when he was depressed or anxious. Learning strategies for coping with anxiety and depression also made him feel more empowered.

In addition, the belief was explored that the voices were powerful because if they said something, it must be true:

> The voices said 'you killed your mother'. The circumstances of his mother's death were explored. Ralph had believed that he should have done something to stop his mother's illness from cancer. However, he accepted that he and his family had done all they could to help their mother through her illness. Ralph concluded that she had died of an illness (cancer) and that he was in no way responsible for her death.

> The voices called Ralph a pervert. However, there was no evidence to support this claim. Ralph had never taken advantage sexually of another person; moreover, he had been the victim of abuse as a child, not the perpetrator.

> The voices called Ralph evil. Ralph defined an evil person as someone who would not feel guilty about, but would enjoy, physically or emotionally hurting someone; and would not help other people in any way. There was no evidence that Ralph was evil but there was much evidence that Ralph was kind and caring and disliked upsetting people.

Such evidence cast doubt on the truth of what the voices said, leading Ralph to conclude that the voices were liars and not to be trusted. Consequently, he concluded that he did not have to believe the voices when they threatened or said unpleasant things about him or others.

The following belief was also explored: that because the voices said things frequently, sometimes getting louder, they should be obeyed. This was challenged by asking him to consider whether saying 'you are a pink giraffe' to someone over and over again would make this statement true. Ralph concluded that just because something is said repeatedly does not automatically mean it is true or that he should act on it.

Gradually, Ralph began to believe that he could choose whether or not to believe what the voices said, and he could choose whether or not to act on their commands.

Exploring beliefs around compliance with or resistance of command voices

The advantages and disadvantages of acting on commands were explored. Ralph concluded that he would resist commands to kill or harm others either because he did not want to harm the person or because of the negative consequences, such as being imprisoned. He began to believe that the voices relied on him to act for them and that they could not physically make him act. Ralph identified that he was more vulnerable to obeying commands to harm or kill himself when he was depressed. A plan for managing his behaviour at such times was developed.

Reducing appeasement

During therapy, Ralph chose to resist more serious commands to harm himself or others, but he did respond to commands to 'get out of bed', which was viewed as an appeasement or safety behaviour. Ralph was encouraged to resist these minor commands to see if the supposed consequences ensued. They did not.

Exploring beliefs about meaning and identity

Ralph believed he was being persecuted for past misdemeanours. An alternative explanation was proposed, namely the notion that stressful events in childhood and adolescence had triggered the development of Ralph's mental health problems. Links were made between Ralph's relationship with the voices and his relationship with his abuser. As a child, Ralph had felt powerless to act against the abuser; similarly, Ralph had perceived himself to be subordinate to the voices, in the same way as he had been to the abuser. However, therapy was enabling him to become more assertive with the voices and with significant others; for example, Ralph was learning that he could make choices about his behaviour that might contradict the voices' commands. Ralph began to describe various situations with friends, family and staff in which he had been able to assert himself: for example, he initiated a move from a flat into supported housing because he felt that this would be beneficial for his mental health; he began to actively seek support from trusted others whenever he felt distressed by the voices or other events; and he started to talk more openly about his experiences with trusted others, no longer feeling ashamed to do so.

Outcome

The Voice Power Differential Scale (VPDS; Birchwood *et al.*, 2000) and the control and distress scales of the Psychotic Symptom Rating Scales (PSYR-ATS: Haddock *et al.*, 1999) were administered before and after the intervention. The VPDS measures the power differential between voice and voice hearer on five-point scales, with regard to overall power and a number of related characteristics. The PSYRATS measures the severity of a number of dimensions of auditory hallucinations and delusions, including amount and intensity of distress associated with these symptoms.

A major reduction in distress was observed, accompanied by a shift in the power balance favouring Ralph, as shown in Table 3.2. The results indicate

Table 3.2 Summary comparing pre- and post-therapy measures for Ralph (1–5 scales)

Measure		Pre-therapy	Post-therapy
Voice power differential[1]	Power	5 (voices much more powerful)	3 (we have same amount of power)
	Strength	5 (voices much stronger)	3 (we are as strong as each other)
	Confidence	5 (voices much more confident)	3 (we are as confident as each other)
	Knowledge	5 (voices much more knowledgeable)	3 (we have same amount of knowledge)
	Harm	5 (voices more able to harm me than I, them)	5 (voices more able to harm me than I, them)
	Superior	5 (voices greatly superior)	5 (voices greatly superior)
Control over the voices[2]		3 (I have some control but only occasionally)	1 (I have some control on the majority of occasions)
Distress[2]		1 (very distressing)	3 (neutral: neither distressing nor comforting)
Beliefs			
Resistance/compliance		5 Compel me to obey them	3 Fairly distracting
Identity of dominant voice (percentage certainty)		Voice of his abuser: 100%	Voice of his abuser: 50%
Meaning of the voices		Persecuted for past events (100%)	Voices mixing up his thoughts (50%)

[1] Voice Power Differential Scale (VPDS).
[2] Psychotic Symptom Rating Scale (PSYRATS).

that the majority of targeted beliefs about the voices had significantly changed by the end of therapy. Ralph believed that he had more control over the voices and was as powerful as them. He had not felt compelled to act on serious commands to harm himself or others, and he no longer believed that he was being persecuted. In addition, the findings indicate that Ralph was somewhat less distressed by the voices post-therapy, although he was still upset by the fact that he continued to hear malevolent voices. With regard to the voices' identity, some doubt had been cast on Ralph's belief that one of the voices was that of his abuser, although he remained partially convinced. Ralph felt that he had benefited from having the opportunity to talk about the voices, in terms of learning how to cope with them and learning that he was able to question what they said and stand up to them.

Chapter 4

Tom

In this and the following six chapters we describe in detail the application of CBT for CH to a range of individuals suffering from command hallucinations, starting with Tom. In all cases the therapist was Dr Sarah Byrne, the first author. The cases have been chosen from the 19 participants in our trial (Chapter 11) to represent the wide range of types and levels of difficulty experienced by men and women from differing backgrounds and ages. Thus we have not selected our 'best' cases but a range from the more to the less successful, in order to provide the clinician with a realistic picture of the challenges involved in the application of CBT for CH. The presentation of each case follows the protocol described in Chapter 3, although, as the reader will see, this is done with considerable flexibility and care, to accommodate to the idiosyncratic needs of the individuals. The reports begin with some brief background information about the individual, followed by the main sections of assessment and intervention (subdivided to describe the key tasks and issues addressed), and concluding with an account of the outcome, with data from the key measures showing the progress (in most cases) of each individual. Recommendations for continuing care are also included in every case. We begin with Tom.

Tom's background

Tom is a 49-year-old man who reported first hearing a voice in his twenties following the death of his father, and subsequently at the time of his mother's death: both parents died of cancer. He experienced remission from the voices for almost 25 years, until recently, when he began to hear a voice daily.

Stage 1: Assessment stage

During the initial assessment, Tom reported hearing one male voice, which said two things only: 'go in the road' and 'set yourself alight'. Tom experienced the voice as very distressing and frightening, and he often felt compelled to obey it. At the time of assessment, Tom reported hearing the voice at least twice a day, particularly during the evenings when he was alone. He found that listening to music and taking his prescribed medication helped to reduce the effects of the voice somewhat.

Beliefs about power and control

According to the Voice Power Differential Scale (Birchwood *et al.*, 2000), Tom believed that the voice was more powerful, much more confident and knowledgeable than him; much more able to harm him than he was able to harm it; and he respected the voice more than it respected him. However, he rated himself as being much stronger than and superior to the voice.

According to Tom, the voice was powerful because he believed that:

- the voice was in control of his life
- he had no control over when the voice occurred or stopped
- the voice knew all about him and could read his mind
- the voice knew what it was doing
- the voice tried to make him harm himself.

Beliefs about compliance/resistance

In response to the voice, Tom described how he had walked into a main road on four occasions, had once set fire to a chip pan and, on another occasion, had tried to burn his shirt; furthermore, he had partially complied by standing on the kerb on several occasions. When he resisted the voice, he described feeling better but tense, fearing that he might be harmed by the voice in some way. Tom predicted that he was 90 per cent likely to obey the voice at the time of assessment and in the future, thus posing a significant risk to himself.

At the time of the assessment, Tom was rated as 'high risk of acting on the voices' commands, with likely harm to self', and he was rated as 'reporting high levels of distress associated with the commands'.

Beliefs about identity

Tom did not know the identity of the voice, although he thought it might have been someone he had known in the past.

Beliefs about meaning

Tom believed that he was being punished by the voice, although he did not know why. He believed that the voice was trying to make him harm himself.

Target behaviours

The main compliance behaviours targeted for intervention were acting on commands to walk in the road and set himself alight.

Stage 2: Intervention stage

Engagement in therapy

From the outset, Tom was keen to participate. He was well motivated to talk about the voice, to explore various issues and to try homework tasks.

Challenging beliefs about control over the voices

Supported by the therapist, Tom developed a range of coping strategies that helped him to have more control over the voices. Distraction techniques worked particularly well, including listening to music and focusing on the words of familiar songs; keeping busy with housework, cooking, gardening and various social engagements; watching interesting TV; phoning a trusted member of his family; going for a short walk and taking prescribed medication.

Sometimes Tom found that the voice stopped for a while if he told it to 'shut up' or 'go away' in a firm voice (out loud when alone or to himself when in company).

Exploring beliefs around compliance with or resistance of command voices

Tom's beliefs around feeling compelled to obey the voice's commands were challenged. For example, Tom had feared that 'something might happen' if he resisted the voice's commands: further exploration revealed his fear that the voice would command him to do something more harmful, making him feel shaky and anxious. The evidence for this was explored: Tom concluded that, when he had resisted the voice, there was no evidence of more harmful commands, and although he often felt a bit shaky he also felt relieved. Through Socratic dialogue, Tom began to develop the belief that the voice was not a physical object and, therefore, could not physically harm him. He began to realise that the voice relied on him to act and could do nothing if he chose not to; that the voice could only frighten him with words and was powerless to act.

Furthermore, Tom had feared the convincing, stern way in which the voice spoke. This was challenged by questioning whether saying something in a particular way necessarily makes it true or right, and whether telling someone to do something means that they must always act. Tom was asked if he would hop around the Day Centre if told to do so in a stern way by the therapist: he was certain that he would not. Tom concluded that he could choose whether or not to believe what the voice said, and whether or not he acted on its commands.

In addition, the advantages and disadvantages of acting on the commands were explored: Tom began to realise that obeying the voice put him in danger, made him feel distressed and the voice did not stop for long; but resisting the voice meant that no harm came to him and, if the voice got louder and more aggressive, he could cope by standing up to the voice or using distraction techniques. He concluded that he was better off resisting the voice's commands.

Reducing appeasement

Tom described often appeasing the voice's command to 'go into the road' by standing on the kerb. In therapy, we talked through this process in detail. Tom observed that the voice was worse when he was alone in his flat, particularly at night when he was preparing to go to bed. In response to the command voice he would get up and go outside, then he would either stand by the kerb or go into the road: usually his neighbours would return him to safety.

Through discussion we developed an alternative sequence of events for Tom to try: at bedtime he could play music to help him relax in preparation for sleep and to focus his attention away from the voice. He would try to resist the voice's command in the knowledge that no harm would befall him.

Gradually he began to resist the voice, at first getting to the edge of the pavement before resisting, firmly telling himself 'Go back in the house!' Then be began resisting leaving his flat, by saying firmly 'No, I'm not going in that road' and listening to relaxing music. Finally, he was able to ignore the voice by continuing with an activity despite the voice's command. Subsequently, Tom reported not hearing the voice at all.

Exploring beliefs about the power of the voice

By trying the various coping strategies described earlier, Tom began to believe that he had more control over the voice. This was used as evidence to support an emerging belief that he had as much power as the voice.

Subsequently, challenging the belief that the voice could make Tom harm himself gave further support for the view that the voice is far from powerful.

By mid-therapy, Tom reported that the voice had stopped (and it didn't return for the remainder of therapy). He explained that he had refused to obey the voice, saying firmly 'If you're so powerful, do it yourself! I'm not!' He felt able to say this because he no longer believed that the voice could physically harm him or make him act. Following this, Tom continued to believe that, if the voice returned, he would be able to stand up to it and he would know how to cope better with it.

Exploring beliefs about meaning

During therapy, the origins of Tom's voice were explored: there seemed to be a clear link between significant life stressors and the emergence of the voice. The stress/vulnerability model was proposed as a possible explanation for the presence of the voice. This model suggests that people may have a greater or lesser predisposition to psychotic experiences or other physical/mental health symptoms, which are triggered by higher or lower numbers of stressful events experienced. In Tom's case, bereavement seemed to have first triggered the voice on two occasions, 25 years earlier. In recent years, a build-up of events seemed likely to have triggered the voice again: redundancy, followed by excessive alcohol use; the death of his fiancée and the subsequent death of a girlfriend; and finally working in excess of 80 hours a week. Tom began to question the belief that the voice was a punishment, instead concluding that the voice was a response to extreme stress in his life.

Stress management was introduced with a view to minimising the impact of future stressors on Tom's mental health. Strategies included: being aware of his limits (with a view to achieving a reasonable balance between doing too much and too little); setting realistic expectations around family contact (i.e. making decisions about how much family contact was reasonable to expect); and graded practice (i.e doing things in gradual stages).

Mid-therapy, Tom experienced a traumatic incident whereby he was mugged and threatened with a knife. He coped extremely well by using all available support networks, including staff, family, church members and the therapist. This was used as evidence of his ability to cope with severe stress in a positive and proactive way, challenging his previous view that he was too fragile to cope with adverse events. Tom's own resources to cope with stress were emphasised, in addition to seeking support from others.

Bereavement issues pertaining to his parents were explored: Tom wrote a letter to his father expressing previously unspoken thoughts and feelings; and, through discussion in therapy, Tom concluded that he was not to blame for his mother's death. Furthermore, Tom's fear of 'breaking down' again if any further significant others died, and ways of preventing this happening, were explored.

Exploring beliefs about identity

Tom had surmised that the voice may have been someone he had known in the past, although he could not identify whom. The therapist proposed a possible alternative explanation for his experience of hearing a voice, namely as misattributed inner speech or automatic thoughts (see Nelson, 1997: 184–187). Everyday examples of how the brain can misinterpret information were presented. Tom seemed to find this explanation feasible and helpful as an alternative to the idea that the voice was an actual person. It also helped to explain his original beliefs that the voice knew all about him and could read his mind.

Other issues addressed in the therapy

- Tom described a number of incidents in which he had had disagreements with people: he tended to feel upset, worried and sometimes extremely depressed after the event. A problem-solving approach was used to encourage him to be more effectively solution-focused, instead of emotion-focused. Tom reported finding this approach helpful in resolving difficulties and reducing symptoms of anxiety and depression.
- Another problem arose around Tom's expectations of his family: he described becoming upset or angry if they didn't phone him at least every other day. Discussion about how much family contact was reasonable to expect led to the conclusion that such frequency of contact was unrealistic and likely to lead to Tom feeling disappointed: a more realistic compromise of once or twice a week was agreed.
- Events that triggered feelings of depression in Tom were explored and framed in terms of CBT 'vicious circles'. Ways of breaking these depressive mood cycles were identified.
- The belief 'nobody cares for or loves me' was explored and challenged: Tom concluded that there was much evidence to the contrary and none to support this belief.
- The 'brag slot' was introduced to help Tom focus on daily positive achievements, rather than his tendency to focus on negative events. Tom agreed to set aside some time each afternoon to review all the things he had achieved or enjoyed in the past 24 hours (e.g. making someone laugh, doing some housework). He found this a very positive exercise, helping him to realise that most days he was capable of achieving something that made him feel good about himself.
- Although Tom lived alone, he had an excellent support network, including family, friends at church, mental health service users and staff. He was encouraged to maintain this network of people, particularly when he felt low or upset. Tom stated that 'a problem shared is a problem halved'.
- Tom expressed an interest in returning to work eventually. He was aware that excessive working hours were detrimental to his mental health: he was encouraged to take gradual steps, perhaps doing voluntary or part-time work initially, and to seek support and advice from trusted others.

Outcome

By the end of therapy, Tom reported that he was no longer hearing a voice and, therefore, he was not feeling distressed by it. He believed that he was 100 per cent in control of the voice, was much more powerful, and would be able to cope even if the voice returned. In addition, Tom developed doubts about the identity of the voice, becoming somewhat convinced that it could be a hallucination triggered by his own brain, rather than coming from another person. Beliefs about the meaning of the voice also changed: pre-therapy Tom believed that the voice was a punishment; by the end of therapy, he believed that the voice was triggered by a build-up of stressors in his life. More generally, Tom seemed to make progress, over six months, in terms of sleeping better and feeling more able to cope with stress and depressed mood.

Pre-therapy and post-therapy measures for Tom are summarised in Table 4.1. The Voice Power Differential Scale (VPDS; Birchwood et al., 2000; Appendix 1 in this volume) and the control and distress scales of the Psychotic Symptom Rating Scales (PSYRATS; Haddock et al., 1999) were administered before and after the intervention. The VPDS measures the power differential between voice and voice hearer on five-point scales, with regard to overall power and a number of related characteristics. The PSYRATS measures the severity of a number of dimensions of auditory hallucinations and delusions, including amount and intensity of distress associated with these symptoms.

The results in Table 4.1 indicate significant positive changes in Tom's beliefs about the power and control of the voices by the end of therapy (data for the 12-month follow-up was not obtained). In particular, post-therapy, Tom believed that he was much more powerful than the voice, that he was able to have control over it and that the voice was not distressing at all.

Table 4.1 Summary comparing pre- and post-therapy measures for Tom

Measure		Pre-therapy	Post-therapy (6-month follow-up)	Post-therapy (12-month follow-up)
Power differential[1]	Power	4	1	No data
	Strength	1	1	No data
	Confidence	5	1	No data
	Knowledge	5	1	No data
	Harm	5	1	No data
	Superior	2	1	No data
Control over the voices[2]		4	0	No data
Distress[2]		4	0	No data

[1] Voice Power Differential Scale (VPDS).
[2] Psychotic Symptom Rating Scale (PSYRATS).

Conclusion

Tom reported that he had really enjoyed the therapy sessions and said that he felt sad to be ending them. In the therapist's view, he had benefited greatly from talking about his difficulties, and learning adaptive ways of coping with them. As Tom stated: 'I'm getting there!'

Recommendations

At the end of therapy, the following recommendations were made by the therapist, for support staff to pursue.

- To encourage Tom to continue engaging in current activities, as well as creating new possibilities, such as resuming employment.
- To support Tom in taking gradual steps in returning to work, perhaps doing part-time work to begin with. Furthermore, he may need assistance in finding a suitable job where he is not put under undue pressure.
- Tom has considered moving to a group home where he will have the company of other people. He may choose to pursue this in the future.
- To use the summary handout provided by the therapist to regularly review their work together, with particular emphasis on Tom's ability to cope with stress and depressive symptoms.

Chapter 5

Joan

Joan's background

Joan is a woman in her late fifties who reported first hearing voices several years ago after a long-term relationship ended. Prior to this relationship she described a difficult marriage to a man who misused alcohol and offered limited support in the upbringing of their children.

Stage 1: Assessment stage

During the initial assessment, Joan was rated as moderately to severely depressed: she reported using alcohol as a way of coping with her difficulties. Joan said that she heard three voices (two male, one female), which she found very distressing. They were described as extremely loud, often shouting and almost continuous.

Beliefs about power and control

According to the Voice Power Differential Scale (Birchwood *et al.*, 2000; Appendix 1, this volume), Joan believed that the voices were much more powerful and confident than her and superior to her; and much more able to harm her than she was able to harm them. She also believed that she respected her voices much more than they respected her. She believed that the voices were much more powerful because:

- she had no control over when they started or stopped
- they knew all about her
- they could read her mind.

However, she rated that she was as strong as the voices and that she and they had about the same amount of knowledge.

Beliefs about compliance/resistance

In addition to being critical of her and abusive, Joan reported that the voices frequently commanded her to harm herself. There was little evidence that she had acted on these commands but she feared that she might act because of the persistent and convincing nature of the voices. However, on three occasions Joan had found herself walking down the middle of the road in the early hours of the morning. She said that she had been unaware of having heard a command to do this but she had heard the voices saying 'we've won, we've won', which she took as evidence of the voices' power to make her comply. As soon as she had realised where she was she had moved to the pavement. Joan reported always resisting commands to 'cut your throat' and 'douse yourself with petrol', despite feeling anxious and panicky. The voices also told Joan to 'jump off a motorway bridge' and although she did not act on this command, on a few occasions she reported that she had prepared to leave the house, but then had decided not to comply by remaining at home. Furthermore, Joan reported that the voices commanded her to 'get rid of other people' sometimes, which she always resisted. At the time of the assessment, Joan was 60 per cent convinced that she would not act on the voices. She said that she did not want to act because she knew that what the voices asked was wrong, although she feared that she might act.

At the time of the assessment, Joan was rated as 'reporting high levels of distress associated with the commands', with 'lower risk of acting on the commands'.

Beliefs about identity and meaning

She did not know who the voices were but believed that she was being punished by the voices, although she did not know why. She believed that the voices were trying to harm her by telling her to do terrible things.

Target behaviours

The main compliance behaviours targeted for intervention were Joan's fears of acting on commands to harm herself or others.

Stage 2: Intervention stage

Engagement in therapy

Joan was keen to participate in therapy but had grave concerns as she had stopped seeing two therapists previously due to the voices' threats to harm them. On one occasion, the voices had commanded Joan to take a knife or hammer to the therapy session and to use it on the therapist, so Joan had not attended again for fear of complying. Consequently, it was crucial for the therapist to convince Joan to give therapy a chance this time around. Promoting the idea of Joan engaging in therapy needed to be handled carefully.

The therapist explained that she was prepared to take responsibility for the voices' direct threats to harm her, if Joan agreed to inform her each time the voices told her to harm the therapist, or if Joan felt the need to appease the voices (e.g. by carrying a knife). The therapist emphasised that it was not her aim to get rid of the voices, rather the aim was to help Joan understand her experience of them, and to explore different coping strategies that other voice hearers have found helpful, with the overall aim of reducing Joan's distress. It was explained that people often feel anxious when they first talk about their personal experiences (including hearing voices), and sometimes their voices seem worse initially (e.g. louder or more aggressive), but, after a few sessions, people tend to feel more relaxed and more able to trust the therapist, and find it helpful to talk about their difficulties. Joan agreed to give this therapy a chance.

Challenging staff beliefs about CBT for CH

Concerns about Joan participating in therapy were also expressed by staff. Joan was a psychiatric inpatient at the time of her referral for CBT for CH, and there were some concerns about her safety and that of others once she was discharged. The therapist acknowledged these concerns but stated that there was no evidence of Joan acting on serious commands to harm herself or others: the only time she had *seemed* to act in response to the commands was when she had walked in the middle of the road at night on three occasions. Concerns were also raised about the risks associated with Joan talking about her voices: some staff feared that talking about the voices could make them worse. Such fears are not uncommon, particularly in staff with a traditional 'medical model' training. Evidence supporting the efficacy of CBT for voice hearers was cited; in particular, it was emphasised that there was no evidence of CBT making voice hearers worse and increasing evidence of the benefits to voice hearers of talking about their experiences and feeling listened to and understood. The therapist agreed to proceed carefully with Joan and to 'back off' if therapy appeared to be causing any deterioration in her mental health. Furthermore, it was felt that disallowing CBT at this stage would give Joan the message that she could not benefit from talking about the voices and learning to cope more effectively with them (thus maintaining a view of self dependent on the support of others). The general conclusion was that Joan could benefit from therapy and that concerns about risk could be alleviated by taking appropriate precautions. It was agreed that Joan would remain an inpatient during the early stages of CBT, to monitor risk and to ensure the availability of appropriate support for her. The therapist arranged for ward staff support to be available to Joan before and after each therapy session. Moreover, Joan said that she felt safer in hospital because the ward doors were locked at night, preventing her from obeying the voices' commands.

Prior to each session, the therapist prepared appropriate safety precautions (e.g. alerting staff that the session was about to commence; sitting near a suitable exit, with access to a panic alarm). Furthermore, at the beginning of each session, the therapist asked Joan to report any threats of harm to herself or others made by the voices, and clarified whether Joan ever felt compelled to act on these commands. Throughout the therapy sessions, there were no instances where the therapist felt that Joan was at risk of acting on commands to harm herself or others.

Once she was discharged from the ward, therapy sessions took place in Joan's local day centre where she could access staff support before and after sessions, and where the therapist had access to a suitable safety procedure. As before, throughout therapy, Joan never behaved in a way that warranted concerns about safety to self or others.

Joan engaged extremely well in therapy; she was keen to talk about her experience of hearing voices, to explore various issues and to try homework tasks. Whenever she was unable to attend, she always cancelled and rearranged. When her attendance became more erratic near the end of therapy, it was because she was reluctant to end the sessions.

Challenging beliefs about control over the voices

Over the sessions, Joan began to develop a variety of ways of coping with the voices. Distraction techniques included talking with or being in the company of trusted others, and keeping active (e.g. regularly attending the day centre, gardening, reading, watching interesting TV, listening to music, doing housework and going for short walks). Sometimes Joan was able to ignore the voices by focusing her attention on something that interested her.

In addition, Joan found that the voices sometimes stopped for a while if she told them to 'shut up' or 'go away' in a firm voice (out loud when alone or to herself when in company). Joan also tried shadowing the voices: repeating word for word what the voices said, with the aim of reducing their frequency. Furthermore, Joan reported feeling less depressed and anxious when she took her prescribed medication regularly.

Exploring beliefs around compliance with or resistance of command voices

Beliefs were challenged around Joan's fear that she might act on commands to harm herself or others, as follows.

1   Joan had feared that the voices would hurt her in some way if she

resisted. The evidence for this was explored. Joan reported that she felt anxious and panicky when she resisted, and the voices got louder. However, there was no evidence of her ever being *physically* hurt by the voices: the voices often made empty threats to harm her if she resisted but there was no evidence of them having ever carried out these threats in all the years she had heard them. Through Socratic dialogue, Joan began to consider alternative beliefs: that the voices were not physical objects and, therefore, could not physically harm her; that the voices relied on her to act and could do nothing if she chose not to; and that the voices made empty threats and never acted on them.

2   Joan had also feared that the voices would harm the therapist if Joan attended therapy sessions. A technique recommended by Nelson (1997) was used, which involved the therapist issuing a direct challenge to the voices to harm her. First the therapist summarised why she did not think that the voices could do as they threatened. Then the therapist challenged the voices directly to cut off her little finger during the session, rather than telling Joan to harm her. The therapist made it clear to Joan that she was taking full responsibility for the challenge and for any harm that might come as a result. Initially, Joan was anxious about the proposal but she agreed to allow the therapist to try it.

The outcome was that Joan reported that the voices became silent, and nothing happened to the therapist's finger. Subsequently, the therapist showed Joan her little finger at the beginning of each session: Joan would appear pleased. This powerful technique provided convincing evidence that the voices were not all-powerful. Furthermore, there was no evidence of the therapist or the previous two therapists coming to any harm from the voices. It was highlighted that the voices seemed to rely on Joan to act for them despite the fact that she did not want to harm anyone. It was concluded that the voices were unable to physically harm the therapist or anyone else: what they did was to frighten Joan by making idle and empty threats that they were unable to carry out themselves.

3   Joan had also felt compelled to comply with commands because of the persistent, convincing way in which the voices spoke. This was challenged by asking her to consider whether saying 'you have green hair' to someone over and over again would make this come true. Joan concluded that just because something is said repeatedly does not automatically mean it is true, and just because the voices tell Joan to do something, this doesn't mean that she has to act.

4   Joan revealed that she felt distressed because part of her was convinced that the voices might act on their threats. The evidence was reviewed:

- The voices were not able to physically harm.
- Joan did not act because she did not want to.
- The voices never reacted physically when Joan chose to resist.

- The voices relied on Joan to act but she always chose not to.

In addition, the voices' content was discussed: the therapist asked Joan how she would feel if the voices said 'douse yourself in rosewater' (instead of petrol): Joan said that she would not feel frightened at all. Joan concluded that it was the words used by the voices that upset her: she began to believe that just because the voices said unpleasant things, this did not mean that they could act on them or that they had the power to make her comply. Gradually, Joan began to believe that she could choose whether or not to believe what the voices said, and she could choose whether or not to act on their commands.

The advantages and disadvantages of acting on the commands were explored: Joan was aware that obeying the voices could put her in danger and make her feel distressed, and that they would be unlikely to stop for long, if at all. However, resisting the voices meant that no harm came to her or others, and although she often felt anxious initially, this anxiety gradually subsided and she sometimes felt good for resisting. Furthermore, while the voices often got louder and more persistent when she resisted, she knew that they could not act and that she could use coping strategies to help reduce her distress. Joan concluded that there were more advantages in resisting the voices' commands.

Evidence of the likelihood of Joan obeying commands to harm herself or others was explored. It emerged that Joan had never actually complied with direct commands: the only time she had *seemed* to act in response to the voices was when she had found herself walking in the middle of the road at night. An alternative explanation for this behaviour was proposed: Joan may have been sleepwalking. Any risk of this happening again was resolved by making sure that her external doors were locked at night, so that she could not unwittingly leave the house in the middle of the night.

Exploring beliefs about the power and control of the voice

By trying the various different coping strategies described earlier, Joan began to believe that she had more control over the voices. This was used as evidence to support an emerging belief that she had as much power as the voices.

Subsequently, challenging beliefs that the voices could make Joan harm herself or others gave further support for the view that the voices were not as powerful as she had previously thought. Gradually, Joan began to believe that she had more control because she chose to resist the voices' commands.

Gently mocking the voices, by showing them to be cowards for making empty threats and relying on others to do their dirty work, also helped to emphasise the voices' lack of power and to give Joan a further sense of control over them.

Exploring beliefs about meaning

Pre-therapy, Joan believed that she was being punished by the voices, although she did not know why. However, during therapy, the stress/ vulnerability model was proposed as a possible alternative explanation for the development of Joan's mental health difficulties, including hearing voices and feeling depressed. This model suggests that people may have a greater or lesser predisposition to psychotic experiences or other physical/mental health symptoms, which are triggered by higher or lower numbers of stressful events experienced.

Relationship difficulties seemed to be a key contributing factor for Joan. In particular, the ending of a long-term relationship seemed to have triggered her voices. Furthermore, it is likely that alcohol misuse played a role in maintaining her difficulties.

By the end of therapy, Joan reported being 100 per cent convinced that the voices had been caused by a build-up of stresses in her life, rather than being a punishment.

Exploring beliefs about identity

Joan was unsure about the identity of her voices: sometimes she thought that they came from inside her head; other times she felt convinced that they came from outside. The therapist proposed a possible alternative explanation for her experience of hearing voices, namely as misattributed inner speech or automatic thoughts (see Nelson, 1997: 184–187). Everyday examples of how the brain can misinterpret information were presented.

By the end of therapy, Joan had some doubts that the voices were actual people, and was 50 per cent convinced that her brain may have misinterpreted internal sounds as coming from outside.

Other issues addressed in the therapy

Linking the voices and depressed mood

Through discussion, Joan began to observe that the voices were much worse when she was feeling depressed, and when she was unoccupied. The therapist explained how depression can be understood in terms of a vicious cycle of negative thinking, avoidant behaviours and low mood. Ways in which Joan could break out of this vicious cycle were explored, as follows.

1   It was highlighted that Joan sometimes chose to avoid social contact when she was feeling low in mood but that such avoidance was likely to exacerbate the problem, as she would have more time alone to focus on her negative thoughts. Joan was encouraged to talk to people she could

trust about how she was feeling (e.g. staff, family or friends) rather than withdrawing into herself. Furthermore, Joan agreed to allow unplanned visits from trusted others, rather than avoiding answering the door. Also, Joan said that she would endeavour to go to the day centre even when she was feeling ambivalent about attending. The importance of maintaining a good support network was emphasised.

2   Activity scheduling was introduced: that is, planning daily activities that gave Joan a sense of achievement and/or pleasure. It was emphasised that having some structure to each day would give Joan a sense of purpose, and could distract her from the voices, as well as improving her mood. The therapist also liaised with Joan's adult children with a view to supporting Joan with activities such as swimming and shopping.

3   A problem-solving/CBT approach was used to encourage Joan to identify what had triggered a specific episode of low mood, and to identify alternative explanations and possible solutions.

4   It was observed that the voices' content often reflected Joan's own negative automatic thoughts, and that the voices never said positive or comforting things. Challenging both Joan's negative thinking and the voices' content was explored by working through specific examples in therapy.

The advantages and disadvantages of using alcohol as a way of coping with the voices

Joan reported that she would sometimes binge on alcohol as a way of 'blotting out' the voices and negative thoughts about the past or present. The costs and benefits of this coping strategy were explored and recorded for Joan as outlined in Table 5.1.

Joan concluded that using alcohol was more costly than beneficial. Triggers and alternative ways of coping were identified. In addition to strategies described earlier in relation to coping with the voices and depressed mood, Joan came up with the following ideas: limiting the amount of money she had available to buy alcohol or saving up all the money she would normally spend on alcohol and using it to buy something really nice for herself; buying non-alcoholic drinks or treating herself to chocolate, instead of alcohol; trying new things, like swimming or a college course; starting later in the day if she did choose to drink alcohol; reminding herself that often she was able to refrain from drinking alcohol for days or weeks. Further discussion revealed that Joan found it difficult to resist drinking alcohol at times and she believed that, for her, it was better to abstain from alcohol completely rather than trying to drink in moderation. It was recommended that additional support from an alcohol service might be beneficial.

Table 5.1 Advantages and disadvantages of alcohol use as a coping strategy for Joan

Advantages	Disadvantages
• Blots things out (i.e. the voices, thinking about the past) for a maximum of 2–3 hours	• The voices and thoughts return, and are often worse. Stops me from coping with the voices and thoughts in other, more beneficial ways
• Temporarily improves my mood	• I feel more depressed afterwards (because alcohol acts as a depressant, and counteracts the effects of my antidepressant medication)
• Helps to pass the time	• Stops me from doing other activities that might be give me a sense of achievement or enjoyment
• Sometimes tastes nice	• Sometimes tastes stale. Unpleasant side effects, such as my mouth feeling dry (dehydration)
	• I often drink in secret for fear of upsetting my children. This makes me feel ashamed. Also, I feel ashamed for letting myself down by drinking excessively
	• Long-term/excessive alcohol use can cause damage to parts of the body, including the liver and heart

Other distressing experiences

In addition to hearing voices, Joan described other distressing experiences, including: seeing people on the walls; feeling that she was being watched and ridiculed; and believing that people could read her mind. These beliefs were explored in turn, and alternative explanations considered. Consequently, Joan seemed partially convinced that people could not read her mind and that she might be experiencing visual hallucinations triggered in her brain by stress. Ways of coping with these experiences were discussed.

Relationship issues

Relationship issues were explored: specifically, Joan seemed to be experiencing grief around the loss of her most recent relationship. More complex issues relating to her childhood were not explored due to time limitations, although Joan said that she would like to discuss such issues in future therapy. A referral for psychotherapy was recommended, after a break from therapy of at least six months, to further explore issues around negative childhood experiences and past relationships.

Finally, Joan expressed an interest in participating in part-time voluntary work and was encouraged to pursue this with the help of her support worker.

Ending therapy

Joan's attendance became increasingly erratic near the end of therapy (she cancelled four appointments). Discussion revealed that Joan was reluctant to end the sessions, because she believed that she had benefited from talking about the voices and was concerned that she would revert to feeling powerless against the voices without regular reinforcement once therapy ended. The therapist acknowledged Joan's feelings but emphasised her strengths and ability to cope. In addition, ways in which she could maintain the positive effects of the therapy were explored. Joan was given a detailed summary of their work, which she was encouraged to review regularly by herself and with her support worker. She was also encouraged to continue attending the day centre regularly as a way of coping with the voices and gaining valuable support from trusted others.

Outcome

By the end of therapy Joan reported feeling better in herself more generally: she had noticed that she was finding it easier to get up earlier, that she was more communicative with people and that she was doing more each day. Furthermore, Joan reflected that talking about the voices had helped her to feel less ashamed and more open about the experience of hearing voices. She said therapy had enabled her to see the voices 'in a different light', as less powerful, making her feel less threatened by them. She reported being 100 per cent convinced that the voices could not harm her or anyone else, relying on her to act for them; and 100 per cent convinced that she would not comply. Furthermore, she rated herself as having 95 per cent control over the voices.

Pre-therapy and post-therapy measures for Joan are summarised in Table 5.2. The Voice Power Differential Scale (VPDS; Birchwood *et al.*, 2000) and the control and distress scales of the Psychotic Symptom Rating Scales (PSYRATS; Haddock *et al.*, 1999) were administered before and after the intervention. The VPDS measures the power differential between voice and voice hearer on five-point scales, with regard to overall power and a number of related characteristics. The PSYRATS measures the severity of a number of dimensions of auditory hallucinations and delusions, including amount and intensity of distress associated with these symptoms.

The results in Table 5.2 indicate a significant change in Joan's beliefs about the overall power of the voices over a 12-month period: from believing that the voices were much more powerful than her to believing that she was more powerful than the voices. Furthermore, at 12-month follow-up, she believed that the voices were unable to harm her and that she was superior to the voices. Beliefs about the strength, confidence and knowledge of the voices did not change significantly. Finally, results at 12-month follow-up confirm that

Table 5.2 Summary comparing pre- and post-therapy measures for Joan

Measure		Pre-therapy	Post-therapy (6-month follow-up)	Post-therapy (12-month follow-up)
Power differential[1]	Power	5	3	2
	Strength	3	3	3
	Confidence	5	4	5
	Knowledge	3	5	5
	Harm	5	4	2
	Superior	5	1	2
Control over the voices[2]		4	4	2
Distress[2]		4	4	3

[1] Voice Power Differential Scale (VPDS).
[2] Psychotic Symptom Rating Scale (PSYRATS).

Joan was feeling more in control of the voices, but that she was still distressed by them.

Conclusion

Verbal feedback from Joan and the above results indicate that Joan had benefited from talking about the voices and other issues, as well as learning adaptive strategies for coping with the voices, depression and alcohol misuse.

Recommendations

At the end of therapy, the following recommendations were made by the therapist, for support staff to pursue.

- To encourage Joan to continue engaging in current activities, as well as creating new possibilities, such as part-time voluntary work.
- To offer Joan continued support in coping with depression: in particular, giving her space to discuss her feelings and look at coping strategies.
- To consider referring Joan for psychotherapy after a break from therapy of at least six months, to enable her to further explore issues around negative childhood experiences and past relationships.
- To monitor Joan's use of alcohol as a coping strategy and to consider a referral to an alcohol service for further management of this problem.
- To use the summary handout provided by the therapist to regularly review their work together, with particular emphasis on the voices' *in*ability to physically harm and Joan's ability to resist the voices' commands.

Chapter 6

Tony

Tony's background

Tony is a 40-year-old man with a history of psychosis since his 20s. He reported first experimenting with alcohol and cannabis when he was 15, and described what appeared to be his first visual hallucinatory experience a year later. In his late teens, Tony developed an interest in rock music and, as part of the music culture he was in, started experimenting with a variety of illegal drugs, including speed, LSD and acid: as a result he described having many 'strange' experiences, including visual and auditory hallucinations. He reported first hearing voices in his early twenties. Around the same time, two of his friends died in road traffic accidents, his grandfather died and the band he was playing in disbanded. Furthermore, he reported that his girl-friend decided to have an abortion without involving him in the decision. At this time, Tony described becoming paranoid: acute anxiety was diagnosed. Subsequently, he was admitted to a psychiatric hospital, and was in and out over the next few years. When Tony was in his late twenties he took an overdose in response to voices telling him to kill himself and another hospital admission ensued. Since then he has lived with his parents while receiving support and treatment from community mental health services.

Stage 1: Assessment stage

During the initial assessment, Tony described hearing many voices, both male and female, with a young male voice being most dominant. He said that the voices occurred almost continuously and were extremely loud, often shouting. He reported that the voices frequently commanded him to harm himself: for example, telling him to 'kill yourself', 'cut your wrists', 'hang yourself' or 'cut it', which he interpreted as meaning his body. They were often critical of him, e.g. saying 'you are rubbish', and hostile, e.g. swearing at him or calling him unpleasant names. Unsurprisingly, he found the voices extremely distressing. Tony found that the voices were worse during the day.

Beliefs about power and control

Tony believed that the voices were all-powerful, and that there was nothing he could do to reduce their intensity. According to the Voice Power Differential Scale (Birchwood *et al.*, 2000), he believed that the voices were much more powerful, stronger, confident and knowledgeable than him, and much superior to him; much more able to harm him than he was able to harm them; and he respected the voices much more than they respected him. He believed that the voices were 100 per cent powerful because:

- he had no control over when they occurred or stopped
- he could not avoid listening to them
- the voices were very loud
- they were sent from God.

Despite reporting no control over the voices, Tony said that he was able to converse with them: for example, when a voice said 'kill yourself', Tony would sometimes reply 'I'm not going to kill myself'.

Beliefs about compliance/resistance

Tony reported complying with the commands on one occasion, in his late twenties, when he took an overdose in response to the voices telling him to kill himself: he said that he had not wanted to die but had felt compelled to obey the voices. However, he denied ever self-harming (e.g. cutting) in response to the voices. At the time of the assessment, Tony was 100 per cent convinced that he would not act on commands to harm himself or others, unless he believed that God wanted him to. However, he expressed fear that God might tell him to kill himself and then he would feel compelled to act.

At the time of the assessment, Tony was rated as 'reporting high levels of distress associated with the commands' with 'lower risk of acting on the commands'.

Beliefs about identity

Tony was 100 per cent convinced that one of the voices sounded like a male family member, and that another sounded like an unknown young male. In addition, he sometimes believed that the voices were messengers from God.

Beliefs about meaning

Tony believed that the voices had been sent by God to punish him for giving up playing the guitar in his twenties.

Target behaviours

The main compliance behaviours targeted for intervention were acting on commands to harm or kill himself.

Stage 2: Intervention stage

Engagement in therapy

Initially, Tony appeared very anxious and seemed ambivalent about attending therapy sessions at his local health centre, preferring to be seen at home for the first appointment. His support worker also expressed doubts about his attendance away from home.

Tony described how, for many years, he had been unable to go out at all, locking himself in his room for much of the time. More recently, however, he had begun to venture out a little, visiting his grandmother and two friends. His anxieties about getting to the health centre were explored. Apart from being unsure which bus to catch, Tony reported that his main concerns were feelings of paranoia that he often experienced while waiting for the bus and during the journey. However, there was evidence of recent occasions when he had managed bus and train journeys. Ways of managing his concerns were explored: for example, Tony found that listening to relaxing music on a personal stereo or looking out the window helped to reduce his anxiety while on the bus. Tony's recent successful journeys and coping strategies were highlighted to encourage him to try attending therapy at the health centre. Also, advantages of meeting at the health centre were emphasised, including private, therapeutic space, without the risk of interruption or others overhearing, as well as an opportunity to get out of the house and meet other people.

The next session, Tony arrived early at the health centre, rewarding himself with a cup of tea. He seemed pleased with his accomplishment and was further praised by the therapist. They reviewed his journey in some detail and he agreed to continue attendance at the health centre. Over time, his anxieties around travelling on the bus began to subside and the therapist observed that he was decreasingly anxious on arrival. By mid-therapy, he reported looking forward to meeting at the health centre.

Throughout the sessions, Tony engaged extremely well in therapy and was well motivated to talk about the voices, explore various issues and try some homework tasks. The therapist tried to make the meetings rewarding for Tony by spending part of the session discussing topics of interest to him: for example, talking about his holiday or their mutual interest in music.

Challenging beliefs about control over the voices

Supported by the therapist, Tony developed a range of coping strategies that helped him to have more control over the voices. Tony learned that he was often able to ignore what the voices were saying by focusing his attention away from them and concentrating on something else. Tony was very interested in a variety of different music styles, and found that listening to music was a useful distraction technique (especially using a personal stereo), although at times he found silence just as relaxing, despite hearing the voices. Other distraction techniques included: talking with or being in the company of trusted others; keeping himself busy (e.g. mowing the lawn, walking the dogs, going to the pub with a friend, attending bible study).

Watching the TV or listening to the radio sometimes helped but, at other times, Tony reported hearing voices through them: when this happened he managed by switching the TV/radio off and doing something else. Sometimes Tony was able to switch off from the voices for a while simply by thinking of something else.

Tony found that the voices also stopped for a while if he told them to 'leave me alone' or 'go to hell' in a firm voice (out loud when alone or to himself when in company).

For Tony, external sound sometimes triggered the voices, such as cars or motorbikes driving past the house, the kettle boiling, aeroplanes or people talking: he reported that the louder the sound, the louder the voices became. Some voice hearers have found that putting an earplug in one ear helps to reduce the volume of the voices (see Nelson, 1997). Tony seemed ambivalent about trying this strategy but tried it once: he found it disorienting and decided not to try again. Instead, he found that being in a quieter area where there was less traffic helped, such as his grandmother's house.

Exploring beliefs around compliance with or resistance of command voices

At the beginning of therapy, Tony was 100 per cent convinced that God was telling him to kill himself: he believed that the voices were messengers from God. Further exploration revealed that this belief was based on Tony hearing the voices say 'up to heaven' and 'that's up': which he interpreted as meaning that he should kill himself.

Through Socratic dialogue, Tony began to doubt this interpretation, and to doubt whether the voices were anything to do with God at all. Further Socratic questioning led Tony to doubt the reliability of a number of assumptions that he had made, as follows.

- Tony began to doubt whether God would want him to kill himself. He questioned how God could be telling him to kill himself on the one hand,

and then also be responsible for the power that came over him, stopping him from killing himself. (At such times, he described how he was unable to physically move, so could not act on commands to harm or kill himself.)

- According to Tony's religious beliefs, God is forgiving and wants everyone to repent their sins; he also believed in the Ten Commandments, which include: 'Thou shall not kill'. Tony concluded that it was very unlikely that God would want or encourage people to kill themselves, no matter what they had done (in his case, giving up playing the guitar).
- Tony also began to question why, if God wanted his life to end, this hadn't happened at the time when Tony took the overdose or since. Tony recalled how he had, on occasions, challenged God to kill him but nothing had happened.
- He began to question the voices' threats: if they were so powerful, why did they seem to expect him to harm himself? Why hadn't they harmed or killed him themselves? Through Socratic dialogue, beliefs were challenged around whether the voices were able to harm Tony physically. He began to consider alternative beliefs:

1   That the voices were not physical objects, and only something physical, like a knife or a bullet, could harm his physical body; therefore, the voices could not physically harm him.
2   That there was no evidence of the voices physically harming him; the fact that Tony was still alive, many years after taking an overdose, suggested that they were unable to carry out their threats.
3   That the voices relied on him to act for them but were powerless when he chose not to obey them.
4   That all the voices could actually do was talk loudly, in a nasty way, making empty threats (although Tony admitted to feeling nervous when they made such threats).

Tony concluded that the voices were not as powerful as he used to think.
- Furthermore, the reliability of the voices was put into question. Tony began to observe that often the voices gave contradictory messages: for example, sometimes they said that God wanted him to kill himself; at other times they said that God would not want him to kill himself. As a result, Tony began to distrust what the voices said and began to wonder whether they were just winding him up.
- The belief that Tony should obey the voices because they told him to was challenged by asking him to consider whether saying 'you have green hair' repeatedly to someone would make this come true. Tony concluded that just because something is said in a convincing, loud or aggressive way, this does not necessarily mean that it is true or right. He began to realise that he had the right to decide whether or not to (a) agree with or believe what the voices said, and (b) act on their commands. Tony was

also encouraged to question what people in general say, and to try to make his own decisions: for example, he reported that he had stopped playing the guitar because other people had told him to, rather than out of choice.

- During assessment, Tony had said that he would obey commands only if God told him personally; however, he began to doubt how he would know for certain whether it was God's command or the voices winding him up or his brain 'playing tricks' (discussed later).

Exploring beliefs about the power of the voice

By trying the various different coping strategies described earlier, Tony began to believe that he had more control over the voices. This was used as evidence to support an emerging belief that he had as much power as the voices.

Subsequently, challenging beliefs that the voices could make Tony harm or kill himself, and casting doubt on the identity and reliability of the voices, gave further support for the view that the voices were not as powerful as he had previously thought. At the beginning of therapy, Tony had believed that the voices were powerful because they stopped him from leading a normal life. Evidence gathered across the sessions challenged this belief: for example, Tony had proved that he could confront his anxiety and feelings of paranoia by using the bus in order to attend weekly therapy sessions at the health centre, and by regularly visiting friends and family.

Furthermore, he had been able to enjoy a week's holiday away from home; he was learning to cope successfully with the voices; and he was learning that he was able to choose when it came to the voices' commands. Rather than staying in his room and waiting for something to happen, Tony concluded that he was going to get on with his life as best he could, in spite of his unpleasant hallucinatory experiences.

Reducing appeasement

Pre-therapy Tony reported sometimes appeasing the voices' commands by saying 'I'll do that later', believing that this would satisfy them in some way. However, as he began to believe that the voices were powerless to make him act, he began to stand up to them by firmly saying things like 'No, I'm not going to do that', rather than trying to appease them.

Exploring beliefs about meaning

During therapy, the origins of Tony's voices were explored: there seemed to be a clear link between significant life stressors and the emergence of the voices. The stress/vulnerability model was proposed as a possible alternative explanation for the development of Tony's mental health difficulties, including hearing voices, other hallucinatory experiences and extreme anxiety. This model suggests that people may have a greater or lesser predisposition to psychotic experiences or other physical/mental health symptoms, which are triggered by higher or lower numbers of stressful events experienced.

Key contributing factors identified were: the use of illegal drugs in young adulthood (particularly those with a hallucinatory effect) combined with life stressors such as three bereavements within 18 months, as well as many previous losses that emerged during therapy; and relationship issues (particularly relating to his girlfriend's decision to have an abortion). During therapy, Tony described the hallucinatory effects he had experienced when taking various hallucinogenic drugs as a young adult (e.g. acid tablets and magic mushrooms). At the time, he had been 100 per cent convinced that these experiences were real, but later realised that what he had seen and heard were not real but were visual and auditory hallucinations. Tony also talked openly about some of the current unusual experiences he endured regularly in therapy and other situations. Links were made between present and past experiences: increasingly, he began to consider that current experiences were also hallucinatory (visual, auditory and tactile) rather than real.

Tony began to question his belief that God was punishing him for giving up playing the guitar, instead considering an alternative explanation: that the voices may have developed due to a combination of the many stressful events in his life and ingesting hallucinogenic drugs. Nonetheless, the distress of experiencing such frequent negative hallucinations and the confusion about which experiences were real or not were acknowledged by the therapist.

Stress management, as well as education around a healthy, balanced lifestyle, were introduced with a view to minimising the impact of current stressors on Tony's mental health. Strategies included: breathing and relaxation exercises; reducing his intake of stimulants, such as tea, coffee, alcohol and cola, to more moderate levels; taking appropriate prescribed medication to help reduce agitation and anxiety; being aware of his limits (not doing too much or too little); problem solving; and maintaining a good support network. Tony's own resources to cope with stress were emphasised, in addition to seeking support from others. At the end of therapy, further support with anxiety management was recommended with his support keyworker.

Exploring beliefs about identity

As mentioned above, Tony began to question whether the voices were real people/messengers from God, or whether they were triggered by a combination of hallucinogenic drugs and extreme stressors. The therapist proposed a possible alternative explanation for his experience of hearing voices, namely as misattributed inner speech or automatic thoughts (see Nelson, 1997: 184–187).

Everyday examples of how the brain can misinterpret information were presented. In addition, Tony described experiences that he clearly identified as 'brain mistakes': for example, on one occasion he recalled feeling utterly convinced that some animals were talking to him, only later realising that this was unlikely and probably a hallucinatory experience.

By the end of therapy, Tony was doubtful that the voices came from God and was 50 per cent convinced that they could be hallucinations triggered by his own brain.

Other issues addressed in the therapy

- Tony seemed to have a tendency to focus on negative events occurring in the news, as well as in his own family; this often resulted in his feeling anxious and depressed. Ways of managing these feelings were explored using a CBT framework, and a problem-solving approach was used to encourage him to be more effectively solution-focused rather than emotion-focused. As there was a tendency for Tony to ruminate about problems, in therapy it was important to acknowledge his feelings and concerns, but then to redirect discussions to minimise rumination. For example, in one session Tony was expressing concern that he had left the taps running at home: he was unable to think about anything else. The therapist talked through events leading up to Tony leaving the house; following discussion he concluded that it was very unlikely that he had left the taps on. Tony decided not to return home and the focus of therapy was redirected.
- The advantages of keeping active were emphasised: preventing boredom; providing daily structure; reducing low mood; helping to quieten the voices; increasing social opportunities. In particular, Tony planned to develop his music interests further, with help from his support worker.
- Tony reported having blaspheming thoughts about God or Jesus that he believed triggered hallucinations. A cognitive ABC model (e.g. Chadwick *et al.*, 1996) was used to explore this: it was identified that having an intrusive thought led to Tony feeling anxious, which may have triggered a visual hallucination. Thus feeling anxious about blaspheming triggered the hallucinatory experience, rather than the blasphemous thoughts themselves. Education about intrusive thoughts was introduced, including normalising the experience of intrusive thoughts, and exploring the difference between having such thoughts and acting on them.
- The belief that other people could read Tony's mind and know his intrusive thoughts was challenged, using a technique described in Nelson (1997).
- On occasions, Tony expressed frustration around his life being somewhat limited in terms of work opportunities, money, relationships and independence. Due to time limitations these issues could not be fully explored in therapy: further exploration post-therapy was recommended.

It was also suggested that Tony might benefit from developing his independent living skills with a view to living more independently in the future, and that living in a quieter environment (away from a busy main road) might be beneficial, due to the fact that Tony's voices were often triggered by loud external noise, such as cars or motorbikes.

Outcome

At the end of therapy, Tony continued to report feeling distressed by the threatening nature of the voices but said that he was more equal in power to them most of the time. He still felt unable to control voice content but did believe that he had control in terms of choosing when to disagree or resist them, and in terms of using helpful coping strategies. Tony continued to be vulnerable to feeling highly anxious about specific events, such as leaving the family house unattended, but he was learning to confront this anxiety rather than avoid it.

More generally, over the six months, Tony had made progress in terms of regularly attending the health centre; being less anxious before and during therapy sessions; increased sociability; and increased reported levels of activity.

Pre-therapy and post-therapy measures for Tony are summarised in Table 6.1. The Voice Power Differential Scale (VPDS; Birchwood *et al.*, 2000; Appendix 1, this volume) and the control and distress scales of the Psychotic Symptom Rating Scales (PSYRATS; Haddock *et al.* 1999) were administered before and after the intervention. The VPDS measures the power differential between voice and voice hearer on five-point scales, with regard to overall power and a number of related characteristics. The PSYRATS measures the severity of a number of dimensions of auditory hallucinations and delusions, including amount and intensity of distress associated with these symptoms.

Table 6.1 Summary comparing pre- and post-therapy measures for Tony

Measure		Pre-therapy	Post-therapy (6-month follow-up)	Post-therapy (12-month follow-up)
Power differential[1]	Power	5	4	5
	Strength	5	4	5
	Confidence	5	4	5
	Knowledge	5	4	3
	Harm	5	3	4
	Superior	5	4	4
Control over the voices[2]		4	4	4
Distress[2]		4	3	3

[1] Voice Power Differential Scale (VPDS).
[2] Psychotic Symptom Rating Scale (PSYRATS).

The results in Table 6.1 indicate no significant changes in Tony's beliefs about the power and control of the voices by the end of therapy and at 12-month follow-up: he continued to believe that they were much more powerful than him and that he had little control over them, and he found them very distressing.

Conclusion

Tony reported that he had enjoyed the sessions and was sad to be ending them. Despite the lack of significant change in the data post-therapy, as described above, the therapist believed that Tony had benefited greatly from talking about the voices, and learning adaptive strategies for coping with them. Tony seemed to be learning to get on with life in spite of hearing unpleasant voices, saying 'we all have a right to live'. Furthermore, his anxiety levels, in general, seemed to have reduced and there was evidence to suggest that he was becoming increasingly active. As Tony stated, attending therapy had 'broken the ice a lot'.

Recommendations

At the end of therapy, the following recommendations were made by the therapist, for support staff to pursue.

- To encourage Tony to continue to engage in current activities, as well as creating new possibilities, such as the opportunity to share his music interests with others and to go out more.
- To offer Tony continued support with anxiety management.
- On occasions, during therapy, Tony expressed frustration around his life being somewhat limited in terms of work opportunities, money, relationships and independence. Further exploration of these issues was recommended.
- To develop Tony's skills and self-confidence around living more independently for future purposes.
- Tony's voices were sometimes triggered by loud external noise, such as cars or motorbikes driving past his house; therefore, living in a quieter environment was suggested.
- To use the summary handout provided by the therapist to regularly review their work together, with particular emphasis on Tony's ability to stand up to the voices and to get on with his life in spite of them.

Chapter 7

Naomi

Naomi's background

Naomi is a 24-year-old woman who reported first hearing a voice when she was 13. She described having taken some unknown 'drugs' after which she experienced a voice talking to her for one day only. A year later she said that she began to hear several voices, which were much louder and more distressing: she experienced these voices as frightening because of their nasty content. Following the onset of these voices, Naomi reported threatening someone with a knife, resulting in admission to a psychiatric hospital where she remained for the most part until the age of 17.

Naomi described a difficult childhood in which she witnessed physical violence between her parents. She was reportedly beaten by her mother and raped at seven years by an adult known to her. At the age of eight, Naomi said that she was referred to a child specialist because of her behaviour. She described how she had found it difficult to communicate: she would stare at the television and scream if her mother tried to talk to her. In addition, during early adolescence, Naomi reported that her parents separated and, subsequently, her mother had difficulties in coping with her and her younger brother.

Naomi also said that, as a result of finding school work difficult, she misbehaved in secondary school and became an outsider from her peers after being suspended for assaulting a teacher. She said that her parents had been unable to help her academically, because their education had been limited. By the age of 24, Naomi was living in supported housing with other young people with mental health problems.

Stage 1: Assessment stage

During the initial assessment, Naomi described hearing 'hundreds' of voices, both male and female, with a female voice being the most dominant. She reported hearing the voices almost continuously, both inside and outside her head. She described them as extremely loud, often shouting, and said that their content was always unpleasant or negative. She said that the voices frequently commanded her to harm or kill herself (e.g. telling her to 'cut your wrists', 'jump out of windows', 'go in front of cars', 'eat what's in the toilet', 'put hot water on yourself'), and that often they threatened to 'mash' her (i.e. kill her themselves). According to Naomi, the voices were also very critical of her, saying things like 'you are ugly' and 'you are no good'. Unsurprisingly, Naomi said that she found the voices very distressing.

Beliefs about power and control

According to the Voice Power Differential Scale (Birchwood *et al.*, 2000; Appendix 1, this volume), Naomi believed that the voices were more powerful than her, much more confident than her and superior to her, and much more able to harm her than she was able to harm them. She rated herself as being as strong and knowledgeable as the voices and rated 'we respect each other about the same'. She believed that she had some control over the voices, but only occasionally (i.e. most the time they were uncontrollable). She believed that the voices were 50 per cent more powerful than her, because:

- she had very little control over them
- she was unable to stop them talking
- of their attitude and their tone
- the voices made her do things, including harm herself
- the voices could read her mind and commented on things she was thinking
- they knew all about her, and her past
- they made predictions about the future.

Despite reporting little control over the voices, Naomi said that she was able to 'call up' the voices and have conversations with them.

Beliefs about compliance/resistance

Naomi reported that she had complied with some of the voices' commands to harm herself or others on several occasions in the past, including starting a fire, cutting her wrists and legs, taking an overdose and throwing hot water over another person. At those times, Naomi reported feeling compelled to obey the voices out of fear: she had believed that if she resisted, the voices would harm her, and would increase in frequency and in their aggressive, nasty tone. She also reported that she had felt pain in her body if she resisted the voices' commands. At the time of the assessment, however, Naomi reported being 100 per cent convinced that she would *not* act on commands to harm herself, others or property because she believed that it was wrong to do so. Nonetheless, Naomi said that she did comply with innocuous commands, such as 'tidy your room' and 'eat food', about two or three times daily. She believed that it was in her interest to comply with such commands and that their frequency decreased once she complied.

At the time of the assessment, Naomi was rated as at 'high risk of acting on the voices' commands, with likely harm to self or others', and as 'reporting high levels of distress associated with the commands'.

Beliefs about identity

Naomi was unsure about the identity of the voices, although she said that sometimes she believed them to be the spirits of dead people.

Beliefs about meaning

Naomi reported being 100 per cent convinced that the voices had been caused by taking some drugs when she was younger. She also believed that she was being punished for past misdeeds and that the nasty tone of the voices meant that they were trying to harm her in some way.

Target behaviours

The main compliance behaviours targeted for intervention were acting on commands to harm herself or others.

Stage 2: Intervention stage

Engagement in therapy

During the first session, Naomi was reluctant to discuss the voices because she said that they were 'going on at her'. The therapist reminded Naomi that the aim of therapy was to help Naomi understand her experience of hearing voices, and to help her develop some coping strategies that other voice hearers have found helpful, with the overall aim of reducing her distress. The therapist was careful to go at Naomi's pace, exploring Naomi's experience of hearing voices in a gentle, empathic way.

Following this session, Naomi appeared keen to participate. She engaged extremely well, and was well motivated to discuss issues and try homework tasks. However, her attendance at sessions was somewhat erratic and on a number of occasions the therapist arrived for therapy only to discover that she had gone out. Staff tried to ensure that she was around at the time of the sessions, but she would sometimes 'disappear' despite their best efforts. When this issue was discussed in therapy, Naomi would insist that she wished to continue participating and reported finding the sessions helpful.

Challenging beliefs about control over the voices

Supported by the therapist, Naomi began to develop a variety of ways of coping with the voices, enabling her to have more control over them.

Distraction techniques included: keeping occupied (e.g. regularly attending college, going for a walk or out shopping, tidying her room, cooking); talking with or being in the company of trusted others; reading a good book or listening/dancing to music; watching an interesting TV programme or video.

Naomi tried standing up to the voices by disagreeing with what they were saying or by telling them to 'shut up' or 'go away'. However, she found that they would respond by saying nastier and more aggressive things, resulting in Naomi becoming more upset and angry. Consequently, she decided that it was better to ignore them as much as possible, and get on with other things, rather than engage in conversation with them: this way she found that the voices bothered her less.

Gradually, Naomi began to realise that she was able to gain respite from the voices at times when she was fully occupied (e.g. when attending college or when engaged in conversation), thus reinforcing such behaviour.

Mid-therapy, Naomi observed that the voices sometimes began when she was stressed or worried about something. She found that relaxation and/or distraction techniques helped (for example, slowing down her breathing, focusing on smoking a cigarette or going out for a walk).

Exploring beliefs around compliance with or resistance of command voices

The first step to challenging beliefs around compliance/resistance was to cast doubt on the reliability of the voices. If the voices could be shown to be unreliable then the therapist could later argue that perhaps they were less powerful than Naomi had previously believed, and thus not worthy of being obeyed.

Firstly, the belief that 'everything the voices say is true' was questioned. Pre-therapy, Naomi had believed almost everything the voices said, making her feel very distressed and leading her to believe that either they would actually do as they threatened or they could make her do these things. During therapy, evidence for and against the belief 'everything the voices say is true' was explored, as follows.

1   The voices threatened to 'mash' (i.e. kill) Naomi, but this had never happened.
2   The voices would taunt Naomi by saying things like 'your nose is too big' or 'it's ugly'. However, evidence suggested that many trusted others (including her boyfriend) believed that Naomi was very attractive, in both appearance and personality. Similarly, the voices would say that

Naomi smelled bad when she had just had a shower. Naomi concluded that the voices were telling lies about many things. She began to believe that the voices said such negative things just to wind her up and to upset her. This didn't mean that such statements were true.

3   Naomi observed that, most of the time, the voices said negative things about her and what she was doing; they rarely commented on her positive attributes.

4   It was identified that the voices said things that were contradictory. For example, they made comments about Naomi's room being untidy, but when it was tidy they still complained; or they would say 'you're ugly' one minute and 'you're beautiful' the next. Naomi concluded that she couldn't win with the voices, so she would just do what she wanted to do, and agree with what she wanted to agree with.

5   It was noted that the voices tended to repeat themselves often. Naomi described them as being like a 'stuck robot', saying the same things over and over again. She concluded that just because the voices say something again and again, this doesn't make it true or right, and doesn't mean she has to act on it.

Gradually, Naomi began to question the reliability of the voices: she concluded that the voices were unreliable and could not always be trusted. The more she began to doubt the truth of the voices' content, the less she was upset by them, and the easier it was to ignore what they said. She began to realise that just because the voices say something in a convincing or aggressive way, this does not necessarily make it true or right, and does not mean that she has to believe it, agree with it or act on it.

The next step to challenging beliefs about compliance/resistance was to challenge the belief that the voices could harm Naomi or make her harm herself.

•   Through Socratic dialogue, Naomi began to believe that only something physical, like a knife or a bullet, can harm the physical body and, because the voices are not physical objects, they cannot do any physical harm to her.

•   It was acknowledged that the words the voices used and their loud volume could, at times, upset Naomi. Nonetheless, it was emphasised that words alone could not *physically* harm her. Naomi concluded that just because the voices said horrible things, this did not mean they could act on them or that they had the power to make her act on them.

•   It was observed that the voices seemed to rely on Naomi to do what they said. The therapist explored what happened when Naomi chose *not* to act. She reported that she had resisted the voices' commands to harm herself on many occasions and no harm had befallen her as a consequence. Moreover, the voices had never acted when she had chosen to resist. Naomi concluded that the voices could not physically make her comply: in effect, they were powerless to act; all they could do was talk.

- Furthermore, it was observed that, if the voices were going to hurt or kill her, they could have done it a long time ago. Again, this suggested that the voices were making empty threats that they never carried out.
- Naomi reported that on one occasion she had challenged the voices to cut her themselves. They had said they couldn't do it, thus reinforcing the view that they were powerless to act.

Naomi became less fearful that the voices could harm her if she resisted their commands. Consequently, she felt more able to choose when she complied or resisted. For example, she decided that she was happy to comply with some commands when she felt like it, such as 'clean your room', but that she would resist any commands to harm herself or other people. Naomi came to the conclusion that the voices were not as powerful as she had previously thought, and that she was more powerful than she used to believe: she began to consider her relationship with the voices as more equal.

Through Socratic dialogue, the advantages and disadvantages of resisting and obeying the voices' commands were explored. Disadvantages of obeying included seriously harming herself, taking responsibility for the consequences of her actions (for example, possibly being imprisoned for harming another person) and feeling extremely distressed. Advantages of resisting included no harm coming to Naomi or significant others, feeling happier and feeling more in control. Furthermore, Naomi observed that while she often felt anxious initially after resisting the voices' commands, her anxiety gradually reduced, especially when she distracted herself in some way.

Exploring beliefs about the power and control of the voice

By trying the various coping strategies described earlier, Naomi began to believe that she had more control over the voices. This was used as evidence to support an emerging belief that she had as much power as the voices.

Furthermore, by challenging the reliability of the voices, Naomi began to doubt the truth of what they said, which made it easier for her to take less notice of them, thus making her feel more in control and more empowered.

Challenging beliefs that the voices could make Naomi harm or kill herself gave further support for the view that the voices were not as powerful as she had previously thought, and that she was more powerful than she used to believe. Gradually, Naomi began to believe that she had more control because she could decide whether or not to agree with or believe what the voices said, and she could choose whether or not to act on what they said.

Exploring beliefs about meaning

Pre-therapy, Naomi believed that the voices were a punishment for her past misdeeds. During therapy, the stress/vulnerability model was proposed as a possible alternative explanation for the development of her mental health difficulties, including hearing distressing voices, and low self-confidence. This model suggests that people may have a greater or lesser predisposition to psychotic experiences or other physical/mental health symptoms, which are triggered by higher or lower numbers of stressful events experienced.

A number of factors were identified that may have contributed to the development of Naomi's mental health difficulties: traumatic childhood events, such as being raped, physically assaulted and witnessing violence between her parents; problems at school due to learning difficulties; parental separation during adolescence; taking an unknown drug in her teens; and being sexually assaulted. It was acknowledged that Naomi had endured some extreme stressors during her young life. Her current ability to cope and her determination to get on with her life were praised.

By the end of therapy, Naomi reported being 100 per cent convinced that the voices had developed as a result of a build-up of stresses in her life, and that the voices had been triggered by her use of an unknown drug during adolescence.

Stress management, as well as education around a healthy, balanced lifestyle, was introduced with a view to minimising the impact of current stressors on Naomi's mental health. Strategies included encouraging Naomi to know her own limits (e.g. keeping busy but not overdoing it to the point of feeling stressed and anxious); taking things one step at a time, with breaks in between; having a good amount of sleep and eating well; coping with anxiety (e.g. breathing and relaxation exercises; maintaining her intake of stimulants, such as coffee, tea and cigarettes, at moderate levels); learning to problem solve; and taking prescribed medication regularly. Naomi's own resources for coping with stress were emphasised, in addition to seeking help and support from others, and maintaining a good support network.

Exploring beliefs about identity

Pre-therapy, Naomi was unsure about the identity of the voices, although she said that sometimes she believed them to be the spirits of dead people. The therapist proposed a possible alternative explanation for her experience of hearing voices, namely as misattributed inner speech or automatic thoughts (see Nelson, 1997: 184–187). Everyday examples of how the brain can misinterpret information were presented.

Naomi reported that the voices often copied what she said and they seemed to know all about her. This was used as evidence to suggest that the voices might reflect her inner speech or negative automatic thoughts. Gradually,

Naomi began to express doubts as to whether or not the voices were real: while she did not always believe that they were real, they often sounded convincingly real, which she found confusing.

By the end of therapy, she reported being 70 per cent convinced that the voices were experiences triggered by her own brain; but remained 30 per cent convinced that they might be spirits of dead people.

Other issues addressed in the therapy

- Naomi reported experiences of physical sensations as if she had been touched in her private parts. Initially, she attributed such experiences to the voices having sex with her against her will, which she found extremely distressing. However, further discussion revealed that Naomi had been sexually assaulted years earlier. Talking through the events helped Naomi to come to terms with what had happened. In addition, alternative explanations for the physical sensations were proposed, including traumatic memories, symptoms of anxiety and tactile and olfactory hallucinations. Subsequently, Naomi reported feeling less distressed by the experiences.

- Relationships with significant others were discussed. Naomi reported that sometimes she was unable to say 'no' to the demands of others. Ways in which Naomi could be more assertive were explored.

- Naomi's low self-confidence was explored. She tended to describe physical attributes, such as nice hair and being slim, as being of prime importance. Other factors, such as personal qualities and achievements, were highlighted. She was encouraged to identify her personal strengths and to focus on these, rather than her difficulties (as emphasised by the voices). Naomi developed a positive self-talk technique to help her in various situations; for example, she might say 'I can do this!' or 'I can ignore them.' Gradually she began to talk more positively about herself: she concluded that 'people who hear voices can get on with their lives despite the voices: I can too. I have got a future.'

- Naomi observed that the voices were worse during the evenings and at night, when she was trying to sleep. A variety of coping strategies were explored, including talking with staff on late duty, and ways to improve her sleep; in particular, Naomi found it helpful, before going to bed, to smoke less, drink hot chocolate (instead of drinks containing caffeine) and try breathing exercises. She also found that she slept longer at night if she avoided napping during the day.

- Naomi was encouraged to keep active in order to give structure to her day, prevent depressed mood, quieten the voices, reduce boredom and reduce feelings of loneliness by meeting with other people.

Outcome

By the end of therapy, Naomi reported that she continued to hear the voices, but she believed that she had much more control over them. She said that often she was able to ignore them; alternatively she would stand up to them. Moreover, she felt able to resist their commands, especially commands to harm herself or others (only acting when she wanted to, e.g. to have a shower or eat something), because she had learned that the voices could not actually do anything to her. Naomi described the voices as moderately distressing because they were so repetitive and nasty, but said that they bothered her far less than they used to (pre-therapy she had rated them as very distressing).

Pre-therapy and post-therapy measures for Naomi are summarised in Table 7.1. The Voice Power Differential Scale (VPDS; Birchwood *et al.*, 2000; Appendix 1, this volume) and the control and distress scales of the Psychotic Symptom Rating Scales (PSYRATS; Haddock *et al.*, 1999) were administered before and after the intervention. The VPDS measures the power differential between voice and voice hearer on five-point scales, with regard to overall power and a number of related characteristics. The PSYRATS measures the severity of a number of dimensions of auditory hallucinations and delusions, including amount and intensity of distress associated with these symptoms.

The results in Table 7.1 indicate significant positive changes in Naomi's beliefs about the power and control of the voices by the end of therapy, although not all of these were maintained at 12-month follow-up. Post-therapy, Naomi reported that she was much more powerful, confident, and knowledgeable and much stronger than the voices, and much superior to them, she believed that she was much more able to harm them than they were able to harm her (in the sense that they did not like it when she ignored them). At 12-month follow-up she was rating her relationship with the voices as

Table 7.1 Summary comparing pre- and post-therapy measures for Naomi

Measure		Pre-therapy	Post-therapy (6-month follow-up)	Post-therapy (12-month follow-up)
Power differential[1]	Power	4	1	3
	Strength	3	1	3
	Confidence	5	1	5
	Knowledge	3	1	1
	Harm	5	1	3
	Superior	5	1	3
Control over the voices[2]		3	1	0
Distress[2]		4	2	3

[1] Voice Power Differential Scale (VPDS).
[2] Psychotic Symptom Rating Scale (PSYRATS).

more equal in power, strength, ability to harm and superiority. She reported that she was much more knowledgeable than the voices but that they were much more confident. Furthermore, Naomi reported changes in her distress levels over time: from rating the voices as extremely distressing pre-therapy, to only moderately distressing post-therapy, to very distressing at 12-month follow-up. Finally, a significant positive change in beliefs about control over the voices was reported over time: pre-therapy, Naomi reported having only occasional control over the voices; post-therapy she believed that she had some control; and at 12-month follow-up she believed that she was able to control the voices on the majority of occasions.

Conclusion

Naomi reported that she had found the therapy sessions helpful and would miss the opportunity of talking with the therapist. She said that therapy had helped her to make sense of why she hears voices and had made her realise that the voices were not as powerful as she used to believe. Naomi stated: 'I'm learning to cope', 'I'm fighting back', 'I feel more positive'. In addition, Naomi commented that she liked the fact that the summary handout of her work with the therapist was personalised.

In the therapist's view, Naomi seemed to benefit from talking about the voices, and learning adaptive strategies for coping with them. She was learning to get on with life in spite of hearing unpleasant voices, saying: 'I'm gonna do my own thing, what's best for me, not the voices'.

Recommendations

At the end of therapy, the following recommendations were made by the therapist, for support staff to pursue.

- To encourage Naomi to continue engaging in current activities, as well as creating new possibilities.
- To support Naomi in obtaining employment, as she had requested.
- To continue working on Naomi's self-confidence by, for example, encouraging her to focus on her personal strengths.
- To develop her skills and self-confidence around living more independently, as Naomi had expressed the hope of having her own place in the future.
- To use the summary handout provided by the therapist to regularly review their work together, with particular emphasis on Naomi's ability to stand up to the voices and to get on with her life in spite of them.
- To consider further therapy in the future, if appropriate, focusing on past traumatic events.

Chapter 8

Janice

Janice's background

Janice was one of the most complex cases that the therapist worked with during the CBT for CH trial. She was very mentally unwell on several occasions during therapy, resulting in two admissions to the local psychiatric hospital. During each hospital stay she was given a course of electroconvulsive therapy (ECT), which had a significant effect on the CBT, affecting Janice's ability to talk, concentrate and remember for several sessions after each course of ECT treatment.

Other complicating factors included ongoing childcare problems, with social services involved and Janice's parents temporarily caring for her two children; and the fact that both Janice and her husband (Dave) had learning difficulties. More specifically, Janice is dyslexic and had difficulty reading written handouts.

Despite all this, it was felt that Janice was very appropriate for CBT because of the severity of the voices and the high, serious risk of her acting on their commands.

Janice is a 28-year-old woman, married with two young children (aged six and two years). She currently lives with her husband. Her children are on the 'at risk' register and were being cared for by their grandparents throughout the duration of therapy.

Janice described an isolated childhood. Firstly, she did not mix with her peers in primary school: she attributed this to having difficulties with reading and writing, which meant that she had extra teaching support, differentiating her from other children. Secondly, there weren't any children of her own age to play with in her neighbourhood. In addition, Janice described herself as a 'latchkey kid' from the age of 11 years: both her parents worked full-time and Janice regularly arrived home to an empty house. Instead of playing with other children (like her peers) she did washing, ironing and general housework and helped to prepare the evening meal. Janice did have an older brother but she reported little contact with him as he would arrive home later and was often busy doing his schoolwork. Janice said that she had not minded doing household chores as she hadn't known any different, but she had not liked being left alone for up to two hours each afternoon.

Janice reported that her parents had shown little affection towards her as a child: she was rarely cuddled, and she recalled that often her father would reprimand her for doing things wrongly: she did not remember him praising her for good behaviour.

She recalled one incident of physical harm by her father (reportedly he dragged her on the floor by her hair because she hadn't brushed it); she denied any other instances of physical or sexual harm by her family. In addition, Janice had only limited contact with her extended family and was not close to any of them.

At the age of 11, Janice went to a special needs school where she was diagnosed with dyslexia. She continued to have difficulties with reading and writing, and she described how she spent most of her free time looking after the younger children, who treated her as a mother figure. It was here that she met her future husband, Dave.

Janice was a very isolated, lonely child and it seems that the voices developed as a form of friendship when she was 12 years of age. For three years the voices were helpful and comforting companions, advising her on how to cope with everyday things, comforting her when she was upset (for example, saying 'it's all right' or 'you'll be OK'): Janice regarded them as her secret friends.

However, Janice reported that at the age of 15 years she was raped violently by someone known to her: she told Dave (then her boyfriend) but refused to go to the police for fear of what her parents would say. She became pregnant on account of the rape and was encouraged to have an abortion by her family. Her parents assumed that the baby was Janice and Dave's.

Janice blamed herself for all that had happened, and it was shortly after the termination that the voices she heard turned nasty (they have continued to be unpleasant voices ever since).

Stage 1: Assessment stage

During the initial assessment, Janice reported hearing two voices, one male and one female, with the male voice being more dominant. She said that the voices frequently (up to six times daily) commanded her to harm herself and others. For example, they told her 'you have got to burn yourself', 'cut yourself, you know you want to', 'put your head in the oven', 'thump X [one of her children], you know you want to do it, you can't help it', 'go on, do as you are told'. She observed that commands to harm herself were more likely to occur when she was cooking (i.e. near a hot oven or cutting vegetables). The voices were sometimes threatening, saying things like 'I will get her [referring to her daughter] – don't leave her alone in there'. The voices also commented on her behaviour and were often critical of her or swore at her (for example: 'you are not doing that properly', 'you are a stupid cow', 'you're dirty'). Furthermore, the voices sometimes advised her, for example: 'you have got to take your tablets' or told her what she should wear.

She reported hearing the voices almost continuously, often lasting for hours at a time. She said that they sounded like they were inside (not outside) her head, and they were often quiet and mumbled. She described their content as always unpleasant or negative, and she experienced them as very distressing. The voices were causing severe disruption to her life so that hospitalisation was sometimes necessary, although she was able to maintain some daily activities and self-care while in hospital. As one might expect, Janice found the voices very frightening, often feeling upset, panicky and tearful as a consequence.

According to the Calgary Depression Scale for Schizophrenia (Addington *et al.*, 1993) she was rated with moderate depression and hopelessness; severe self-depreciation (feeling worthless more than 50 per cent of the time); pathological guilt (feeling to blame for everything that has gone wrong in her life); and severe early wakening and observed depression. Moreover, she had deliberately considered suicide with a plan but had made no attempts to act.

Beliefs about power and control

According to the Voice Power Differential Scale (Birchwood *et al.*, 2000; Appendix 1, this volume), Janice believed that the voices were much more powerful, confident and knowledgeable than her, much superior to her and much stronger than her. She also believed that the voices were much more able to harm her than she was able to harm them, and she believed that she respected the voices much more than they respected her.

She believed that the voices were 'more than' 100 per cent powerful because:

- she was unable to control them
- they made her do things, such as harm herself and push her children
- they knew about her weaknesses, her fears, bad things she had done in her past
- they knew how to wind her up or make her angry
- they told her what to do frequently.

Janice believed that she had no control over when the voices occurred, and could not dismiss them or bring them on at all. At the time of assessment, her ability to cope with the voices was very limited: on occasions, the voices would stop for a short time if she shouted or ignored them.

Beliefs about compliance/resistance

Most of the time, Janice complied with the voices' commands to harm herself because she was afraid of them. She believed that it was in her interest to comply as she would be harmed if she didn't do as the voices said. She described how she would go into the kitchen and put the oven on until it was hot, then she would put her hand inside the oven and take hold of the shelf until she had burnt herself. Alternatively, she would get a kitchen knife and superficially cut her wrist or arm. She denied wanting to harm herself, saying that she only acted because of the voices' commands. She described a feeling of relief once she had complied as the voices would leave her alone for a few hours, although she knew they would start up again later.

Janice found that if she resisted the voices' commands, they would become more frequent and louder, shouting and screaming, compelling her to act. She described feeling very worried and nervous, as she believed that the voices would go on and on until she gave in. However, there were occasions when Janice was more likely to resist: when she was out shopping or with her parents and children, and when she was feeling better in herself, she felt able to tell the voices to 'get lost' or she would shout and swear at them. In addition, her husband would stop her from cutting or burning herself whenever he could, although Janice said that she would feel upset for fear that the voices would make her act later.

Partial compliance

Janice had tried delaying compliance by thinking 'I'll do it later' but she had found that the voices got more intense and made her feel terrified. Consequently, she tended to choose to 'get it over and done with'. However, there were occasions when she put the oven on but did not attempt to burn herself. In addition, Janice found that using the vacuum cleaner reduced the urge to act, temporarily, although she believed that she would feel compelled to act later. Another appeasement strategy used by Janice was to pick at her wounds as a way of temporarily silencing the voices.

At the time of the assessment, Janice was rated as at 'high risk of acting on the voices' commands, with likely harm to self or others', and as 'reporting high levels of distress associated with the commands'.

Beliefs about identity

Janice was 50 per cent convinced that the voices sounded like her grandparents (now deceased) because of the old-fashioned way in which the voices said things. However, she denied that her grandparents, when they were alive, had ever said such unpleasant things.

Beliefs about meaning

At the time of assessment, Janice reported that she heard these particular voices because she had been unable to cope when she was a child. She was 100 per cent convinced that the voices were trying to harm her in some way, and 100 per cent convinced that they were *not* trying to help her.

Target behaviours

The main compliance behaviours targeted for intervention were acting on commands to harm herself and others, in particular commands to burn or cut herself, and commands to harm her children.

Stage 2: Intervention stage

Engagement in therapy

In order to make it easier for Janice to attend sessions, the therapist arranged to meet with her at her local GP surgery. In the first session, initially, Janice appeared emotionally flat and timid: however, as the meeting progressed, she began to relax and was able to express her feelings quite well. She reported feeling anxious about meeting the therapist: this was acknowledged and normalised.

Janice did not turn up to the second session so, after a short wait, the therapist phoned her at home. This was not the therapist's normal practice but due to the fact that Janice's difficulties often affected her ability to remember things, it was deemed appropriate in this instance. Janice was very tearful, saying that she was due to meet her social worker later that day to discuss putting her children into voluntary care. Janice was clearly upset and said that she felt too unwell to attend the session. However, the therapist suggested that it might help Janice to talk with someone about her concerns.

Exploring current family concerns

They agreed to meet at the GP surgery, focusing on the issue at hand: Janice reported that she was unable to cope with her children at present due to the voices. She said that the voices frequently commanded her to harm her children and, on occasions, she acted on these commands. For example, the voices had said 'Go on, you've got to do it, we won't shut up if you don't', which led Janice to push one of her children into a coffee table. She also reported smacking or thumping the children in response to the voices' commands to: 'hit them, you know you want to do it, you've got to hurt them'. Janice often tried to resist by leaving the room but the voices would get worse, shouting at her, resulting in Janice burning herself. On occasions when she did obey commands to harm her children, Janice tried to hit them less hard because she didn't want to hurt them; however, the voices then said 'you're not doing it properly, you're not hitting them properly'.

Janice told how she was concerned for her children's safety and how she wanted them to have a 'proper childhood'. She worried that her older child had already taken on the role of carer, not wanting to leave her mother to play. Furthermore, she reported that her younger child had delayed speech (and was currently seeing a speech therapist).

At the time, Janice reported finding even simple chores difficult to cope with. She believed that she needed a break from looking after the children in order to catch up on some much-needed sleep and to regain her strength. Her husband, however, wanted the children to remain at home, to be mainly cared for by him. Janice reported that her husband did not fully understand the extent of her difficulties. Moreover, she felt that he would need to take much more responsibility for the children and household chores if the children were to remain with them. Janice's preferred option was to have her parents take care of their children, rather than foster parents, because they were familiar to the children and visiting would be more flexible.

Managing anxiety

In the second session, Janice reported having panic attacks earlier the same day. She described typical symptoms, including difficulty in breathing, hot flushes, shaking, feeling edgy, feeling irritable and upset, and having anxious thoughts relating to her children. In subsequent sessions, the therapist witnessed these symptoms. The first time, it was the end of session three and the therapist was booking a room for the next session. Suddenly Janice began breathing very fast and wailing in a distressed way; she looked really frightened and appeared ready to escape. The therapist calmly directed her to sit down and gently asked Janice to look at her, encouraging Janice to try to slow her breathing. The therapist comforted her and began breathing slowly, counting four in and then six out. Janice began to follow the therapist, gradually slowing her breathing rate down. Once Janice was calmer, they moved to a private room and Janice began to cry, saying she was afraid to go home as her husband was out. The therapist talked this through with Janice and explored how she could cope if her husband was not in: Janice decided that she would have a lie down while listening to the radio with a view to minimising her feelings of anxiety. The therapist gave words of encouragement before Janice left to return home. In the next session, Janice reported that her husband had been at home when she returned and she had felt fine.

Janice had three panic attacks during a subsequent session. Each time, the therapist calmly helped Janice to manage her anxiety, in particular helping her to regulate her breathing. Possible triggers for these episodes were explored.

In addition, the therapist introduced anxiety management information. She was unable to give Janice written information due to her dyslexia. Instead, basic breathing techniques were taught and practised in-session and Janice was given an audio-tape of some breathing and relaxation exercises (which subsequently she reported as being helpful).

Helping Janice to manage her feelings of anxiety was an important part of the engagement phase, contributing to the building of rapport and development of a trusting therapeutic relationship.

For the next few sessions, Janice attended regularly and engaged well in therapy. Although tearful at times, she was able to talk about her experiences of hearing voices. Furthermore, she began to understand the development of her difficulties, describing specific life events that may have contributed to her mental health difficulties.

Electro-convulsive therapy: effects on therapy

After session five, Janice was admitted to the local psychiatric hospital by her consultant psychiatrist and care co-ordinator, due to a reported increase in symptoms of severe depression and in order to monitor her medication more closely. Janice and her family were under considerable stress due to issues relating to the care of her two children; this is likely to have contributed to an exacerbation of the depressive symptoms. In order to maintain therapeutic engagement, the therapist continued to meet with Janice throughout her hospital stay.

As part of her psychiatric treatment plan, Janice was given electro-convulsive therapy (ECT), resulting in short-term side-effects including memory loss, shortened attention span and difficulty in concentrating. Consequently, the therapist decided that CTCH sessions needed to be brief (10–20 minutes) but more frequent (twice weekly). Gradually, weekly sessions resumed, ranging from 30 to 60 minutes depending on Janice's level of concentration and attention. However, progress in consolidating the gains made prior to hospital admission were hampered as a result of ECT treatment, due to the attention, concentration and memory problems.

Nonetheless, Janice managed to attend the majority of her sessions, only cancelling one due to ill health. This suggests that Janice was motivated to continue therapy despite the many complications regarding her case.

Challenging beliefs about control over the voices

Supported by the therapist, Janice began to develop a variety of ways of coping with the voices, enabling her to have more control over them.

Distraction techniques that sometimes helped to focus her attention away from the voices included talking with or being in the company of trusted others (e.g. husband, parents, friends); keeping busy (e.g. doing housework, cooking, gardening); watching something interesting on TV; listening to music; going for short walks; playing computer games.

The therapist observed that Janice would sometimes be distracted by the voices in-session. Exploration revealed that sometimes Janice's husband had to shout at her to draw her attention away from the voices.

Janice began to notice that when she was inactive, the voices were worse and she felt more depressed. The therapist explained how depression can be understood in terms of a vicious cycle of negative thinking, avoidant behaviours and low mood. Consequently, a list of daily activities was drawn up in therapy to encourage Janice to keep active, including going out with her husband or mother, walking the dog, going shopping, household chores, doing a puzzle and playing games with the children. The therapist also requested a referral to a local day centre for Janice. Initially, Janice was anxious about attending but, with support and encouragement, she learned to enjoy meeting other people with similar difficulties to her own and to enjoy some of the activities on offer. In addition to quietening the voices and help-ing break the depressive cycle, other advantages of keeping active were high-lighted, such as giving structure to the day, meeting other people, reducing boredom and feeling less lonely.

A problem-solving approach was also introduced to help Janice feel more in control of the voices. For example, on one occasion, Janice was alone in the kitchen and the voices were commanding her to burn herself. She coped by leaving the kitchen and joining her family in the garden; this helped to dis-tract her from the voices, stopped her from harming herself and made her feel happier.

Sometimes, Janice found that the voices stopped for a while if she or her husband said 'shut up', 'leave me/her alone' or 'go away' in a firm voice (out loud when alone or with Dave, or to herself when in company). By doing this, Janice learned that she was able to stand up to the voices at times, rather than always using distraction to gain control.

Janice also found that she was more able to cope with the voices when she had slept well. Furthermore, taking her medication regularly helped to make her feel less depressed and anxious.

Janice was encouraged to verbalise her view of her power relationship with the voices. She gave the analogy of 'a mouse and a monster': most days Janice was the mouse and the voices were the monster but, occasionally, it was the reverse. Janice described how 'some days it's like having your worst enemy with you, other days I tell them to shut up and go away'. At this stage, the voices were generally seen as more powerful, although Janice was beginning to exert some control over them. It was emphasised that one of the aims of therapy was to help her to develop a more equal relationship with her voices.

Exploring beliefs around compliance with or resistance of command voices

Firstly, the therapist explored with Janice why she sometimes felt compelled to comply with the voices' commands. Janice explained that she acted because of the way the voices said things: in a convincing, stern way. She also feared that the voices would harm her or her family in some way if she resisted their commands. These two beliefs were challenged accordingly.

Challenging the way the voices say things

The belief that one should act just because something is said repeatedly in a dominant tone was challenged. The therapist asked Janice to run around the room shouting 'whoopee!'. Janice laughed and refused. The therapist repeated the request using a more stern, commanding voice: again Janice refused. Similarly, Janice said that she would not act if her husband told her, again and again, to act against her will, including hurting herself. Janice agreed that she was able to choose *not* to act on the commands of others.

Challenging beliefs about harm

However, Janice was still concerned about the consequences of resisting the voices' commands. Thus, the next step was to challenge the belief that the voices could harm Janice or her family, or make her harm herself or others.

- Through Socratic dialogue, Janice began to develop the belief that only something physical, like a knife or a bullet, can harm the physical body; and that as the voices were not physical beings they could not do any physical harm to her or her family.
- It was acknowledged that it was the words the voices used; their stern, authoritative tone; and their persistence that upset Janice and compelled her to act. If the voices had told her to cut an apple in a polite, friendly tone, she would not have felt as frightened. It was emphasised that words alone could not *physically* harm her or her family.
- It was observed that the voices seemed to rely on Janice to do what they said. The therapist explored what happened when Janice chose *not* to act. Janice reported that when she resisted the voices' commands to harm herself, no physical harm came to her or her family. Moreover, the voices had never acted when she had chosen to resist. Janice concluded that the voices could not physically make her comply: in effect, they were power-less to act; all they could do was talk.
- One of the most powerful techniques for disempowering a voice is for the therapist to issue a direct challenge to harm her or him in some way (see

Nelson, 1997: 198–199). Firstly, the therapist summarised why she did not think that the voices could do as they threatened. Then she challenged the voices, directly, to cut off her little finger during the session. The therapist made it clear to Janice that she was taking full responsibility for the challenge and any harm that might come as a result. The outcome was that Janice reported that the voices became silent, and nothing happened to the therapist's finger.

In the next few sessions, the therapist showed Janice that her little finger remained intact. This technique provided convincing evidence that the voices were unable to physically harm; rather they made empty threats.

Challenging the reliability of the voices

The therapist also taught Janice to question the reliability of the voices: if the voices could be shown to be unreliable then the therapist could later argue that perhaps they were less powerful than Janice had previously believed, and thus not worthy of being obeyed. When the voices said something critical about Janice she was encouraged to ask: 'What's the evidence for that?'

In one session, evidence was explored for the voices' accusation: 'you're useless'. Janice was able to identify many strengths, including being a kind and friendly person; showing love and affection to her children; and being a survivor of many difficult times in her life. It was concluded that she was far from useless and, therefore, she could not rely on what the voices said to her.

On a subsequent occasion the voices told Janice she was stupid; this time Janice asserted her view by saying that she was not stupid or daft. Janice reported feeling weird but pleased with her response.

In another session, Janice described how the voices had told her to shut up when she was sitting watching TV: Janice thought this was stupid because she had been silent, so she just ignored them and continued to watch TV.

Gradually, Janice began to question the reliability of the voices: she became more aware that just because the voices say something in a convincing, stern way, this does not necessarily make it true or right, and does not mean that she has to believe or agree with it. Janice was able to conclude that just because the voices were persistent and nasty, this did not mean they had the power to make her act on commands or that they could act.

Using the ABC model

Throughout therapy the cognitive therapy model was demonstrated using specific examples as they arose. The following example aimed to help Janice understand the links between her mood and the process of complying with the voices' commands.

- *Activating events*: Alone at home.
- *Beliefs*: Thinking 'I'm alone' and 'No-one can help'.
- *Consequences*: Feeling anxious, sad and depressed. Behaviour: Sitting doing nothing.

  ○ further negative thoughts, e.g. 'I'm useless'
  ○ feeling more depressed
  ○ voices say 'burn yourself'
  ○ feeling compelled to act on the command
  ○ feeling disappointed in self for acting
  ○ depressed mood increases
  ○ voices continue.

Ways of breaking this process were then explored, including changing behaviours, challenging the beliefs and negative automatic thoughts, and challenging the voices.

Costs/benefits analysis

A costs/benefits analysis of complying with or resisting the voices' commands was conducted. Disadvantages of obeying included seriously harming herself or harming one of her children, an increased risk of her children being taken from her care on a permanent basis, and feeling extremely distressed. Also, the voices did not stop for long, if at all. Advantages of resisting included no harm coming to Janice or her children (even if the voices continued to sound threatening), and feeling more in control and less distressed.

It was emphasised that while Janice might feel anxious initially when resisting the voices' commands, her anxiety was likely to reduce gradually, especially if she distracted herself in some way.

Evidence of resisting command voices

Over the sessions, Janice reported feeling more able to resist the voices' commands. On one occasion she described how the voices had told her to 'get up' in a persistent manner: she was able to resist for half an hour, after which she got up in order to find an alternative way of distracting herself from the voices. Another example of Janice learning to resist the voices was when they advised her on what clothes to wear: Janice was able to say 'I wear what I want'. Such examples were used to support the idea that Janice had a choice regarding compliance with and resistance of the voices' commands.

Later in therapy, Janice reported being able to resist more serious commands to harm herself: she found that, although the voices continued, nothing bad happened to her or her family, and she felt relieved and less worried by the voices.

Exploring beliefs about the power and control of the voices

Challenging beliefs that the voices could make Janice harm herself or others gave support for the view that the voices were not as powerful as she had previously thought, and that she was more powerful than she used to believe. Janice began to believe that she had more control because she could decide whether or not to agree with or believe what the voices said, and she could choose whether or not to act on what they said.

One of the key themes that emerged during therapy was Janice's sense of powerlessness in her life, generally. She described having no control in her life and very limited choices; this contributed to her depressed mood. By enabling Janice to take some control over the voices (using the various coping strategies described earlier), resulting in her feeling more empowered with the voices, it was hoped that there would be a knock-on effect on other areas of her life. Furthermore, Janice was encouraged to have her say during therapy, including feeding back to the therapist how she felt about the progression of the sessions (positive or negative).

The therapist likened Janice's relationship with the voices to any adult relationship: it involved give and take, and choices, such that when the voices, or any adult, told Janice what to do, she could choose whether or not to agree with, or to do, what they said. For example, sometimes Janice was happy to obey the voices when they suggested what she wear (if she agreed), but she was learning that she had the choice to say 'No, I'm not going to do that' when they commanded her to do something she didn't want to do, such as harm herself or another person.

Mid-therapy, Janice described how her 'other self' often disagreed with the voices. She described one situation when one of the voices was trying to take charge by answering all the therapist's questions. Janice managed this by choosing *not* to reply to what the voice was saying because she didn't agree with it. She found the idea of being assertive with the voice rather strange because it was unfamiliar to her, but preferable to being taken over by the voice.

While CBT had introduced the idea of being more assertive with the voices, it was anticipated that further long-term work would be necessary to empower Janice in the wider context.

Exploring beliefs about meaning

At the beginning of therapy Janice believed that the malevolent voices were a punishment for being sexually attacked and having an abortion in her teens. In therapy, Janice was given space to talk through what had happened: she described how she had felt too frightened to tell the police or her parents. Janice said that she now regretted not telling her mother the truth about the baby's origin, as she wanted her mother to know that she would have refused to have an abortion if the baby had been Dave's. She said that she hated herself for having an abortion and that she blamed herself for the rape and for not telling her mother the truth.

The therapist explored the hypothesis that the content of the voices might have reflected Janice's own feelings about herself. Janice confirmed this, saying that it was sometimes difficult to distinguish between herself and the voices: 'It's really eerie trying to work out which part is me and which part is the voices'. Furthermore, it was hypothesised that harming herself might have fulfilled a wish to punish herself for past events: Janice agreed that this was likely. Thus, an important part of the therapeutic process was to work through Janice's beliefs about herself in relation to past traumatic events, and to challenge beliefs around blame and punishment.

During therapy, the stress/vulnerability model was proposed as a possible alternative explanation for the development of her mental health difficulties, including hearing distressing voices and experiencing severe anxiety symptoms. This model suggests that people may have a greater or lesser predisposition to psychotic experiences or other physical/mental health symptoms, which are triggered by higher or lower numbers of stressful events experienced.

A number of factors were identified that may have contributed to the development of her mental health difficulties, including being different from her peers due to her learning difficulties (later diagnosed as dyslexia); lack of parental warmth and affection; feeling isolated due to being at home alone regularly, and not having any local children to play with; lack of supportive relationships within or outside the family while growing up.

It was proposed that lack of nurturing and empathy plus being lonely as a teenager may have triggered the benevolent voices (friendly, helpful and comforting). Then, traumatic events during adolescence are likely to have led to the voices becoming malevolent (nasty and critical of Janice).

Exploring beliefs about identity

Pre-therapy, Janice had said that the voices sounded like her grandparents (now deceased), although she denied that her grandparents had ever told her to harm herself or others, unlike the voices. The therapist proposed a possible alternative explanation for her experience of hearing voices, namely as misattributed inner speech or automatic thoughts (see Nelson, 1997: 184–187). Everyday examples of how the brain can misinterpret information (including the therapist's own experiences) were presented. The therapist also explained how voices can sound like somebody known to the voice hearer (see Nelson, 1997: 184–187).

Over the sessions, Janice began to question whether the voices were a malevolent force external to herself, or whether they were part of herself (i.e. her own internal negative automatic thoughts).

Other issues addressed in the therapy

Absence of the voices

During session four, Janice reported that the voices stopped after she took new antipsychotic medication. Despite their negative content, Janice described missing the voices because they were familiar: she said that she had been used to having them around and was now feeling frightened ('nobody wants to know me now the voices have gone') and lonely in their absence ('I've no-one to talk to now'). Janice's sense of loss and fear of abandonment were discussed, and the advantages and disadvantages of the voices' presence were explored. Janice believed that she was better off without them as they only made her feel distressed, and she believed that she was more likely to get her children back permanently if the voices ceased. However, it was emphasised that it was possible that the voices might return. The therapist explored alternatives to relying on the voices for company, encouraging Janice to extend her support network beyond her husband and family (e.g. attending the local day centre for people with mental health problems).

Predictably, the voices were back by the next session, triggered by a stressful visit to see her children. Janice was encouraged to accept the voices as part of her. She was reminded that learning to cope better with the voices would enable her to feel more in control and less distressed by them. It was emphasised that the experience of hearing voices (positive or negative) did not have to stop her from getting on with her life.

Later in therapy, the voices stopped again for a few days: this was linked to the fact that Janice was feeling better in herself, less depressed and anxious. Again, ways of coping and the possibility of them returning were explored.

Care of the children

Following the meeting with social services regarding the care of Janice and Dave's two children, it was agreed that Janice's parents would become their main carers for the next few months at least, with Janice and her husband visiting twice weekly. Regular reviews of the situation were also agreed.

Bearing in mind that Janice had described her upbringing as less than ideal, the issue of Janice's parents looking after her children was explored. Janice said that her father still got irritable when he was tired; nonetheless, she believed that her parents were more lenient with their grandchildren than they had been with her, and treated them more positively. Furthermore, Janice believed that her father was unlikely to physically harm the children because he had angina and had to be careful about getting too stressed. However, she did express some concerns about her parents treating the children more like objects than little people. Janice talked about her preference for a more 'child-centred' approach to parenting (e.g. allowing the child to take the lead in play whenever possible, and giving both children plenty of physical affection and encouragement). Despite this, Janice and her husband decided that Janice's parents should be carers of their children in preference to unfamiliar foster carers.

Janice's children were a key issue throughout therapy. Janice was concerned that if she didn't get rid of the voices, she might never be able to care for her children full-time. Moreover, knowing that she was unable to care for her children had exacerbated feelings of helplessness. The concept of 'quality time' was raised and the importance of Janice's continued involvement in the upbringing of her children was emphasised, even if she was unable to be their full-time carer. In therapy, Janice was encouraged to increase her ability to cope with the voices and to resist their commands: it was hypothesised that if Janice was feeling more in control of the voices and feeling stronger in herself, it was more likely that her children would be returned to her care.

Systemic work

Systemic work within the wider family context was felt to be appropriate in order to enhance the therapist's understanding of Janice's difficulties, as well as supporting Janice in getting her needs met as fully as possible. By engaging with Janice's family, the therapist also hoped to gain their support for continuation of the therapy.

On three occasions, the therapist arranged to meet jointly with Janice and her husband. A key theme of these meetings was their general lack of control over their lives, with their parents and professionals making the majority of decisions for them. While they understood that the aim of such support was for their benefit, they expressed the view that they would have liked to have been more involved in decisions about their lives whenever possible. This was fed back to those involved in Janice's care: care co-ordinator, consultant psychiatrist and social workers.

The therapist explored Dave's belief that he had no power or control in his relationship with both sets of parents. Dave was able to identify some of his strengths (e.g. caring for his wife and children, being financially independent), and thus challenge the belief that his views were worthless. The therapist likened the parent–child relationship to that of the voice–voice hearer: as children we are expected to obey our parents, but as adults we are able to develop a more equal (adult to adult) relationship where we can choose to agree or disagree with what our parents say; similarly, the aim of therapy is to encourage a more equal relationship between the voice hearer and her voices.

In addition, the therapist offered Dave guidance on how he could support Janice in coping with the voices. Ways in which Dave could help Janice were identified, such as keeping her company; talking to help distract her from the voices; helping her cook dinner when the voices were being threatening;

discouraging her from entering the kitchen unaccompanied when the voices were being threatening or commanding; helping her to identify coping strategies at times when she was finding it difficult to generate her own ideas. He was also encouraged to enable Janice to maintain control wherever possible: involving her in decisions about the house and family, for example. Initially, Dave was sceptical about the success of these strategies, as he believed that medication was the only answer. The therapist challenged this by working through the analogy of Dave's migraines, such that the medication often only worked when combined with relaxation (i.e. lying in a quiet, darkened room). In a similar way, the therapist explained how coping strategies, in addition to medication, could help Janice manage her distressing voices. Reluctantly, Dave agreed to try the strategies suggested, for his wife's sake.

Furthermore, with consent from Janice, the therapist liaised with her care co-ordinator and consultant psychiatrist several times, and attended a ward round near the end of therapy.

Self-harm

The therapist observed that Janice was more able to resist commands to harm others than to harm herself. Exploration revealed that Janice cared less about harming herself because she did not like herself. Janice was encouraged to develop a more balanced picture of herself by identifying her strengths as well as difficulties. Janice found this exercise extremely difficult, but she did manage with support from the therapist.

Other issues

- Janice was given advice about how to cope with setbacks.
- Her own resources for coping with stress were emphasised, in addition to seeking help and support from others, and maintaining a good support network.
- A summary handout of the therapy was presented to Janice on paper and audio tape (due to her dyslexia). A written copy was also given to the care co-ordinator, who was encouraged to go through it with Janice regularly.

Outcome

Originally, Janice was offered 16 sessions of CTCH (as proposed in the protocol of the CTCH research trial). However, in total she met with the therapist individually on 27 occasions, cancelling only one appointment. Unfortunately, the need to treat Janice with ECT hampered progress with cognitive therapy due to attention, concentration and memory difficulties following ECT treatment. This resulted in the need for briefer sessions and nearly twice as many as originally agreed. Furthermore, it was extremely difficult to adhere to the protocol when so many issues emerged in addition to the voices–power relationship.

Despite this, by mid-therapy (session 15), Janice reported hearing the voices less frequently (about once a day) and she was able to resist the voices' commands on the majority of occasions (she reported cutting her wrist superficially only once in the past month). She qualified this by saying 'I'm more sensible now', and 'I'm not daft enough to listen'. Janice described resisting the commands as feeling 'weird but pretty good'.

Janice began to believe that she had some control over the voices most of the time: she said that taking no notice of the voices worked best, although shouting at the voices, having as much stimulation as possible and question-ing the voices also worked at times. Janice explained that she used to listen to the voices because she felt lonely and believed that no-one was there for her, but now she was beginning to feel differently. She described the voices as moderately distressing (compared with 'very distressing' pre-therapy) and she said that she was no longer distressed when she ignored the voices.

Mid-therapy, Janice reported a huge shift in her power relationship with the voices: she rated herself as much more powerful than the voices (whereas pre-therapy the voices were rated as 100 per cent powerful) and much stronger, more confident, more knowledgeable and superior; and she no longer believed that the voices were able to inflict physical harm on her or her family.

Furthermore, Janice no longer believed that the identity of the voices was her grandparents; instead she described them as 'voices from nowhere'. And she no longer believed that the voices were a punishment for past events: she said that she did not deserve to be punished for what had happened in her teenage years.

Subsequently, the gains reported mid-therapy fluctuated depending on Jan-ice's mood. When she was feeling more depressed and anxious (more vulner-able) she found it more difficult to resist commands to harm herself; although, reportedly, she continued to resist on the majority of occasions. Janice said that because she understood more about the voices compared with pre-therapy, she felt more able to resist them.

After session 21, the therapist was informed that Janice had been admitted to the local psychiatric hospital again. The consultant psychiatrist explained that she had been admitted for a further short course of ECT due to depres-sion. As a consequence, CTCH was hampered again due to poor concentra-tion and difficulties in thinking clearly. Furthermore, Janice was unable to engage in very much activity due to the sedative effects of her treatment. A break in therapy for three weeks was agreed, to enable Janice to recover more fully following ECT treatment and to adjust to her new medication regime. At follow-up, Janice and the therapist agreed to end therapy as it was felt that Janice needed to concentrate her energies on becoming well enough to return home permanently and on resolving issues relating to the care of her children.

By the end of therapy, no further gains were reported, although Janice remained motivated to attend therapy sessions despite finding it difficult to keep focused. Janice reported that her meetings with the therapist had allowed her the opportunity to talk to someone who understood her difficulties, particularly in relation to the experience of hearing unpleasant voices, which she found really helpful.

Pre-therapy and post-therapy measures for Janice are summarised in Table 8.1. The Voice Power Differential Scale (VPDS; Birchwood *et al.*, 2000; Appendix 1, this volume) and the control and distress scales of the Psychotic Symptom Rating Scales (PSYRATS; Haddock, *et al.*, 1999) were administered before and after the intervention. The VPDS measures the power differential between voice and voice hearer on five-point scales, with regard to overall power and a number of related characteristics. The PSYRATS measures the severity of a number of dimensions of auditory hallucinations and delusions, including amount and intensity of distress associated with these symptoms.

The results in Table 8.1 indicate some significant positive changes in Janice's beliefs about the power of the voices by the end of therapy, although many of these were not maintained at 12-month follow-up. Post-therapy, Janice reported that she was stronger, more confident and more knowledgeable than the voices, and superior to them; and she believed that she was more able to harm them than they were able to harm her, but she rated the voices as more powerful than her. At 12-month follow-up she was rating her relationship with the voices as more equal in power and strength; but she reported that the voices were much more confident and knowledgeable than her, much superior to her and much more able to harm her than she was able to harm them. Lastly, consistently across the year, Janice rated the voices as extremely distressing and she believed that she had no control over them.

Table 8.1 Summary comparing pre- and post-therapy measures for Janice

Measure		Pre-therapy	Post-therapy (6-month follow-up)	Post-therapy (12-month follow-up)
Power differential[1]	Power	5	4	3
	Strength	5	2	3
	Confidence	5	2	5
	Knowledge	5	2	5
	Harm	5	2	5
	Superior	5	2	5
Control over the voices[2]		4	4	4
Distress[2]		4	4	4

[1] Voice Power Differential Scale (VPDS).
[2] Psychotic Symptom Rating Scale (PSYRATS).

Conclusion and recommendations

Once therapy had ended, the therapist attended a ward round meeting with the hospital consultant psychiatrist to discuss her conclusions and recommendations, as follows.

The therapist concluded that there were indications that Janice had gained some benefits from engaging in CTCH: at times, she was well motivated, insightful and able to think about her difficulties from a psychological perspective. She also began to develop some adaptive coping strategies to help reduce the power and control of the voices, and the distress associated with them. However, given the complex range of Janice's difficulties and the complexities of her treatment package, the therapist concluded that brief cognitive therapy was unlikely to have a sustained impact (as the results in Table 8.1 indicate). In the therapist's view, a long-term multidisciplinary approach would be necessary to support Janice and her family: a referral to assertive outreach services was recommended, as it was felt that a more intensive support system was needed, in addition to her current support from day centre services and social services. Furthermore, Janice and Dave expressed a preference for additional support at home, to minimise the need for Janice to stay in hospital.

In addition, the therapist recommended longer term psychological therapy in the future, with a view to enabling Janice to feel more empowered within her life, and enabling her to further explore and come to terms with past traumatic events. Finally, the possibility of involving Janice in a local voice hearers' support group was suggested.

Chapter 9

Sally

Sally's background

Sally is a 27-year-old woman with moderate learning difficulties. She reported first hearing voices at 12 years when she was resident in a children's home. Sally's mother had been diagnosed with schizophrenia and she was unable to care for her daughter at the time, although Sally visited her regularly.

At the age of 19, Sally reported being sexually assaulted by a man unknown to her. She was very distressed by this but had received good support from staff at her place of residence (supported housing). At 24, Sally recalled 'crying a lot' and being unable to mix with people, as she felt threatened by them. She described herself as 'suffering from a schizophrenic illness'.

Stage 1: Assessment stage

Presentation

Sally presented as a pleasant young woman who talked in a clear but relatively simplistic way. Her level of cognitive understanding was within the moderate learning difficulties range, which meant that communication had to be tailored to her needs. Despite this, Sally was keen to discuss her experiences of hearing voices, she was motivated to engage in the process of therapy and she was able to read and write.

During the initial assessment, Sally described hearing several male voices, with the dominant voice sounding like a man in his twenties. Sally also reported hearing the sound of an unknown baby crying in a distressed way, on occasions. She reported hearing voices from outside (not inside) her head, several times a day. She said that the voices were very loud, they were unpleasant in content and she felt very distressed by them. According to Sally, the dominant voice commanded her to 'stay awake' when she was getting ready for bed, saying 'if you fall asleep at night you will wake up miserable'. The voices also criticised Sally, saying things like 'you are lazy' and 'you are no good'.

Beliefs about power and control

According to the Voice Power Differential Scale (Birchwood *et al.*, 2000), Sally believed that the voices were all-powerful. Specifically, she believed that the voices were much more powerful, confident and knowledgeable than her, that they were much superior to her, that they were much stronger, and much more able to harm her (than she was able to harm them); and she believed that she respected them more than they respected her. Sally rated the voices as 77 per cent more powerful than her because they were able to 'easily lose their temper' and could 'get very loud'; also because they could read her mind; and because they told her things that were frightening.

Furthermore, she believed that she had no control over when the voices occurred, and she could not dismiss or bring them on at all. She described coping with the voices by listening and obeying them, or watching TV.

Beliefs about compliance/resistance

Sally said that, despite wanting to go to sleep, she always complied with commands to 'stay awake' for fear of being harmed or shouted at if she disobeyed. She reported that it was in her interest to comply as 'someone might get angry' and upset her. Sally described feeling unhappy, worried and scared when the voices gave commands. After complying, Sally said that she felt relieved but very tired, and the frequency of the commands remained the same.

In the past, Sally reported that she had complied with commands to 'walk out of home'. However, she believed with 100 per cent conviction that she would not act on commands to harm herself or others because she believed it is wrong to do so. Records showed that Sally had acted out of character five years previously, attacking someone known to her with a knife, although it was not clear whether this had been in response to command voices.

At the time of the assessment, Sally was rated as 'reporting high levels of distress associated with the commands', with 'lower risk of acting on the commands'.

Beliefs about identity

Sally described the dominant voice as a man in his twenties who was tall with short black hair, and always wore a black suit. She said that she did not recognise him as someone familiar to her but said that she feared meeting him.

In addition, she was unsure about the identity of the other voices, although she believed that they must be real people because she heard them from outside (not inside) her head.

Beliefs about meaning

Sally reported that she had no idea why she heard these voices: she believed that they wanted to get at her in some way, although she did not know why.

Target behaviours

The main compliance behaviour targeted for intervention was Sally's compulsion to keep awake at night in response to the dominant voice's command. Although this command was seen as relatively innocuous, there was some concern about Sally complying with more serious commands if the nature of the voices' commands altered.

Stage 2: Intervention stage

Engagement in therapy

Sally engaged well in therapy and was well motivated for the majority of the sessions. However, it was observed that her vocabulary was quite basic and she appeared rather concrete in her thinking. Consequently, the therapist had to check Sally's understanding consistently, rephrasing words or sentences when necessary. Throughout the sessions, the therapist took Sally's level of understanding into consideration; as such, a limited number of key themes were repeated frequently, rather than introducing too many different concepts.

Challenging beliefs about control over the voices

Supported by the therapist, Sally gradually developed a variety of ways of coping with the voices, enabling her to have more control over them. During the day, Sally reported hearing the voices much less, which made her feel happy. The therapist explained, in simple terms, why this may have occurred: when Sally was busy doing other things (e.g. housework, attending college or watching TV) she tended to focus her attention away from the voices, not listening to them as much. Sally was encouraged to continue keeping busy as a way of taking her mind off the voices. Furthermore, techniques enabling her to stop listening to the voices at bedtime were explored. Sally found the following techniques helpful: listening to relaxing music on her personal stereo; writing down her thoughts in a personal diary; making a hot milky chocolate drink; talking to someone she trusted (e.g. a member of staff);

reading quietly to herself; and avoiding stimulants in the evening, including cigarettes, tea and coffee.

An alternative way of gaining control over the voices was also suggested, namely, to confront them directly. As Sally was not a very assertive person, initially she found this difficult but, with practice, she learned to stand up to the voices, sometimes, by telling them to 'stop talking' or 'be quiet' in a firm way. She was encouraged to say this out loud if she wanted (when alone) or in her head (when other people were around).

Exploring beliefs around compliance with or resistance of command voices

The first step to challenging beliefs around compliance/resistance was to cast doubt on the reliability of the voices: if the voices could be shown to be unreliable then the therapist could later argue that perhaps they were less powerful than Sally has previously believed, and thus not worthy of being obeyed.

Pre-therapy, Sally believed almost everything the voices said without question, making her feel very distressed and leading to compliance with the commands. During therapy, Sally was encouraged to question the truth of what the voices said. For example: the voices upset Sally by saying: 'your brother is no good'. The therapist worked with Sally to explore the evidence for and against this statement. Sally described her brother as kind, hard working and a good father to his children; there was no evidence to suggest that he was 'no good'. She concluded that the voices were telling a lie as she believed that her brother was a good person.

In another example, Sally reported that the voices frequently told her that she was useless. Sally was encouraged to ask herself: 'Am I really useless?' She was able to identify many strengths, such as attending college, helping friends and being able to cook and do household chores, which led her to conclude that she was not useless but was able to do many things.

The therapist used these examples to suggest that just because the voices say something, this does not mean that it is true and does not mean that Sally has to believe it or agree with it. As therapy progressed, Sally became more adept at questioning the voices and asserting her own viewpoint, which often conflicted with that of the voices. Sally also learned other ways of dealing with the voices when they told lies, including: (1) saying firmly to them (out loud or in her head) 'No, that's not true' or 'That is a lie!'; (2) taking no notice of what they said; and (3) talking to her mother or a trusted member of staff about it.

Gradually, Sally began to question the reliability of the voices: she concluded that the voices often told lies and could not always be trusted. The more she began to doubt the truth of the voices' content, the less she was upset by them, and the easier it was for her to ignore what they said.

The next step was to challenge the belief that Sally could be harmed if she disobeyed the voices.

- It was acknowledged that what the voices said and their loud volume could, at times, upset Sally. Nonetheless, it was emphasised that words alone could not *physically* harm her. Sally concluded that just because the voices said such things in a convincing or aggressive way, this did not mean that they had the power to harm her.
- It was observed that the voices seemed to rely on Sally to do what they said. The therapist explored what happened when Sally chose *not* to act. For example, Sally liked to have a good wash every morning. Sometimes the voices would say 'you are lazy, you should wash more'. If the voices said such things in the evening Sally took no notice and carried on with what she was doing. Alternatively, she would say, firmly, 'I'm not lazy, I do wash enough!' Sally began to realise that nothing happened to her as a result of ignoring the command or standing up for herself. Moreover, although the voices regularly commanded Sally to 'stay awake' at night, she always fell asleep eventually and no harm came to her as a consequence. It was concluded that the voices rely on Sally to do what they say but if she chooses not to, they cannot make her comply: in effect, they are powerless to act; all they can do is talk.
- Sally also began to realise that the voices did not stop even when she did comply. She concluded that she might as well do what she wanted to do rather than what the voices told her to do.

Gradually, Sally became less fearful that the voices could harm her if she resisted their commands. Consequently, she felt more able to choose when she complied or resisted. For example, she decided that she was happy to comply with commands such as eating more at teatime, but that she would resist commands to 'get up' if she believed that it was too early.

Exploring beliefs about the power and control of the voice

By trying the various coping strategies previously described, Sally began to believe that she had more control over the voices. This was used as evidence to support an emerging belief that she had as much power as the voices.

Furthermore, by challenging the reliability of the voices, Sally began to doubt the truth of what they said, which made it easier for her to take less notice of them, making her feel more in control and more empowered.

Challenging beliefs that the voices could harm her if she disobeyed them gave further support for the view that the voices were not as powerful as Sally had previously thought, and that she was more powerful than she used to believe. Gradually, Sally began to believe that she had more control because she could choose whether or not to act on what they said.

Exploring beliefs about meaning

Pre-therapy, Sally did not really know why she heard voices, although she believed that they wanted to get at her in some way. During therapy, the stress/vulnerability model was proposed as a possible alternative explanation for the development of her mental health difficulties. This model suggests that people may have a greater or lesser predisposition to psychotic experiences or other physical/mental health symptoms, which are triggered by higher or lower numbers of stressful events experienced.

Again, simple language was used; in this case: 'For some people, voices can start when a person has lots of difficulties in her (or his) life. Some people start to hear voices when things get too much for them, or when they become very upset.'

Vulnerability factors that may have contributed to the development of her mental health difficulties included growing up with a mother diagnosed with schizophrenia (including an increased genetic risk) and, intermittently, having to stay in a children's home as a consequence. Furthermore, being sexually assaulted as a young adult may have triggered her subsequent mental health difficulties.

By the end of therapy, Sally reported that she heard voices due to having lots of difficulties in her life and having schizophrenia.

Exploring beliefs about identity

Pre-therapy, Sally believed that the voices she heard came from outside (not inside) her head. Although she was unsure about the identity of the voices, she had described what the dominant voice looked and sounded like (see Assessment section above).

During therapy, Socratic questioning was used to explore whether or not the voices were real people. Sally reported that she had never seen these people, with the exception of the young man. She observed that she was the only one who heard him and the other voices speak, even when other people were in the same room. She also became aware that all the voices often repeated themselves, like a 'stuck' record. Moreover, they had never physically harmed her, despite her fears. These factors helped to cast some doubt on the origin of the voices.

The therapist proposed a possible alternative explanation for Sally's experience of hearing voices, namely as misattributed inner speech or automatic thoughts (see Nelson, 1997: 184–187). In simple terms, the therapist explained how the brain sometimes makes mistakes or plays tricks on us, giving examples, from her own experiences, of how the brain can misinterpret visual and auditory information. This led Sally to describe an occasion when she had been convinced that she had seen the pop star Madonna, only later realising that she had made a mistake: that she had seen someone that resembled the pop star.

Sally began to consider the possibility that the voices were part of her illness (schizophrenia), triggered by her brain, rather than coming from people external to herself. In the last session, Sally reported that she did not think the voices were real people, rather they came from inside her head.

Other issues addressed in the therapy

- Ways of coping with stress were introduced with a view to minimising the impact of current stressors on Sally's mental health. Strategies included getting a good night's sleep (avoiding stimulants after 8pm, such as drinking tea or coffee and smoking); talking to staff or college teachers about problems or concerns; and taking prescribed medication regularly. Sally's own resources for coping with stress were emphasised, in addition to seeking help and support from others.

- Sally described a few occasions when she saw 'visions' that she knew were not real. For example, Sally thought she had seen a bus coming towards her but when she looked again the bus wasn't there. In therapy, alternative explanations for these experiences were explored. Instead of being frightened by them, she began to accept them as experiences triggered by her brain, and began to feel less bothered by them. It was emphasised that many people hear voices and/or see visions, and are managing to get on with their lives.

- In one session, Sally talked about the unwanted sexual incidents that had occurred in her late adolescence. She reported that staff had been very supportive at the time and had given her advice around preventing any further incidents (for example, saying 'No', not accepting lifts from strangers, running away if feeling frightened). However, further discussion revealed that Sally seemed to associate sexual intercourse with unwanted, non-consenting sexual acts only, rather than within the context of a loving relationship. The therapist felt concerned about Sally's potential vulnerability to further incidents without the appropriate support. A specifically designed programme of further education around sex and social relationships was recommended post-therapy.

- In therapy, Sally was being encouraged to stand up to the voices and assert her own views and choices. This seemed timely, as signs of growing independence were emerging for Sally more generally, such that she was being less compliant and expressing her own views more firmly with staff. For example, Sally raised the possibility of moving into independent, but shared, accommodation. She was enthusiastic at the prospect and staff agreed a plan to teach her necessary skills, such as cooking for herself and budgeting. It was hypothesised that while Sally was a young woman, emotionally and cognitively she seemed to be functioning more as an adolescent.

- Halfway through therapy, Sally began to report feeling unhappy and bored with her current job and ready to move on to something more challenging. Sally said that she wanted to meet new people and learn new things. The therapist agreed to discuss this with her keyworker. Subsequently, it was arranged for Sally to attend college to learn appropriate skills in gardening, with a view to working in this field once qualified. It was emphasised that hearing voices did not have to stop Sally from getting on with her life and developing new skills.
- Assertiveness issues were explored: it was observed that Sally's submissive/compliant role in her relationship with the voices seemed to reflect her position in relationships more generally. Further assertiveness training post-therapy was recommended.
- Sally's keyworker was keen to support Sally as much as possible. Consequently, with Sally's permission, the therapist and keyworker met three times to discuss progress and ways in which therapeutic gains could be made during therapy and post-therapy. The therapist was careful to retain confidentiality as much as possible.
- Near the end of therapy, Sally reported that she had not heard any voices for a few weeks. This was attributed to the fact that Sally was feeling mentally well at the time; she was enjoying her new college course and meeting new people. Sally was encouraged to continue getting on with her life regardless of the presence or absence of the voices.
- A summary handout of Sally's work with the therapist was reviewed and amended in the last few sessions. Sally agreed to read the handout out loud, and her understanding of and agreement with each paragraph was checked; some of the wording was simplified.

Outcome

By the end of therapy, Sally reported that she was hearing the voices less frequently (about once or twice a week) and that she was able to cope better with them using various coping strategies. She now believed that she was a bit more powerful than the voices because she could take no notice of what they said sometimes, and because she was able to stand up for herself against them. However, she rated the voices as stronger and more confident than her because of the way they said things, and because she was not very confident.

Sally believed that the voices could still upset her by talking loudly and saying nasty things, but she no longer feared that they could physically harm her. She began to realise that she did not always have to believe what the voices said, and that she could choose whether to obey or resist their commands. She reported that she complied with commands only if she agreed with them and she was firmly convinced that she would not act on commands to harm herself or others.

Sally described the voices as being part of her illness, rather than real people. She now believed that the voices were coming from inside her head rather than being external forces.

Finally, Sally seemed to be learning to get on with her life despite hearing unpleasant voices, saying: 'life is OK at the moment: I am going to college, where I am meeting new people and learning new things'.

Pre-therapy and post-therapy measures for Sally are summarised in Table 9.1. The Voice Power Differential Scale (VPDS; Birchwood, *et al.*, 2000; Appendix 1, this volume) and the control and distress scales of the Psychotic Symptom Rating Scales (PSYRATS; Haddock *et al.*, 1999) were administered before and after the intervention. The VPDS measures the power differential between voice and voice hearer on five-point scales, with regard to overall power and a number of related characteristics. The PSYRATS measures the severity of a number of dimensions of auditory hallucinations and delusions, including amount and intensity of distress associated with these symptoms.

The results in Table 9.1 indicate significant positive changes in Sally's beliefs about the power of the voices by the end of therapy, although these were not maintained at 12-month follow-up. Post-therapy, Sally reported that she was much more powerful, confident, knowledgeable and much stronger than the voices, and much superior to them; and she believed that she and the voices were equally able to harm each other. However, at 12-month follow-up she was rating the voices as more powerful, much stronger, much more confident, more knowledgeable than her, and superior to her, and much more able to harm her than she was able to harm them. Furthermore, Sally rated the voices as very distressing pre- and post-therapy and extremely distressing at 12-month follow-up. Finally, there was no change in Sally's beliefs about control over the voices: she continued to believe that she had no control over the voices across the year.

Table 9.1 Summary comparing pre- and post-therapy measures for Sally

Measure		Pre-therapy	Post-therapy (6-month follow-up)	Post-therapy (12-month follow-up)
Power differential[1]	Power	5	1	4
	Strength	5	1	5
	Confidence	5	1	5
	Knowledge	5	1	5
	Harm	5	3	5
	Superior	5	1	5
Control over the voices[2]		4	4	4
Distress[2]		3	3	4

[1] Voice Power Differential Scale (VPDS).
[2] Psychotic Symptom Rating Scale (PSYRATS).

Conclusion

Sally reported finding therapy 'interesting and helpful': she said that it had been good having someone to talk to about the voices and that she would miss the therapist. In the therapist's view, Sally had benefited from talking about the voices and learning adaptive strategies for coping with them, and she appeared more self-confident and more assertive in general. In addition, attending college had allowed Sally to develop further by encouraging her independence and learning.

CTCH seemed to coincide well with Sally's developmental stage during therapy. She was being encouraged to stand up to the voices, to question what they said and to allow herself to express her own views (which might challenge the voices), in much the same way as adolescents begin to assert their independence from significant adults.

However, therapeutic gains do not appear to have been maintained at the 12-month follow-up: booster sessions might have been helpful in reinforcing coping strategies and key points learned during therapy, as well as in reviewing her progression regarding the following recommendations.

Recommendations

At the end of therapy, the following recommendations were made by the therapist, for support staff to pursue.

• Despite her learning difficulties, staff were encouraged to enable Sally to be more assertive and independent by allowing her more choices and giving her appropriate responsibilities whenever possible. Assertiveness training was also suggested.

• Encouraging increased independence needed to be balanced with staff awareness of Sally's vulnerability and naivety with regard to relationships. It was felt that she would continue to be potentially vulnerable to further unwanted sexual incidents without appropriate support. An individually tailored education programme, taking account of her learning difficulties and focusing on social and sexual relationships, was recommended as a matter of some urgency.

• Sally's keyworker was encouraged to regularly review the summary handout with Sally in order to reinforce its contents.

Chapter 10

Kevin

Kevin's background

Kevin is an 18-year-old man who lives with his mother and her partner. Kevin first came into contact with child mental health services in his early teens: he was diagnosed with acute anxiety and obsessive-compulsive disorder (OCD) (specifically, he had a compulsion towards hand-washing). A few years later, Kevin was admitted to the adolescent unit of a local psychiatric hospital with symptoms of OCD and hearing voices. He reported that he would wash his hands in response to voices telling him to do so. Kevin described a difficult childhood: he reported witnessing his father's angry outbursts when he was very young, when objects would be thrown aggressively. When Kevin was four years old, his father left the family home and Kevin saw him only a few times subsequently. Kevin was raised for the most part by his mother and maternal grandmother: he described growing up as the only male in the house as difficult at times. In addition, Kevin reported some difficulties with reading and writing at school: he said that he was regularly bullied by other children at senior school between the ages of 11 and 15 years, after which he was moved to a special needs school. Finally, Kevin reported that his grandmother had become ill and later died during his last hospital admission; he described feeling very upset as they had been very close throughout his childhood.

Stage 1: Assessment stage

During the initial assessment, Kevin reported hearing two voices (one male, one female), with the male voice being most dominant. Although he heard the voices several times daily, he said that he was most likely to hear them at night. He believed that the voices came from both outside his head (through his ears) and inside his head. The voices were described as fairly loud (louder than his own voice), with unpleasant or negative content that he found very distressing (for example, the voices said 'you are ugly', 'your mother is evil', or swore at him). Furthermore, Kevin reported that the voices commanded him to harm himself and others (e.g. telling him to 'slash your wrists', and 'hit that person'), as well as telling him to throw things and to wash his hands frequently. Kevin described feeling scared of and worried by the voices most of the time.

Beliefs about power and control

According to the Voice Power Differential Scale (Birchwood *et al.*, 2000; Appendix 1, this volume), Kevin believed that the voices were more powerful and more confident than him, much stronger and much more able to harm him than he was able to harm them. However, he rated himself as being much superior to the voices, and he believed that he and they had about the same amount of knowledge, and that they respected each other about the same.

He believed that the dominant voice was more powerful than him because of the way it spoke to him (sounding realistic, getting louder) and because the voice was able to read his mind.

Kevin believed he had no control over when the voices occurred and was unable to dismiss them or bring them on at all. However, he reported that sometimes the voices seemed less intense when he was reading, painting or listening to music.

Beliefs about compliance/resistance

Kevin reported that he had hit people on three or four occasions in the past (including his mother) in response to the voices. He also said that he had partially complied with commands to slash his wrists on one occasion in his teens, by taking a knife to his wrists but not cutting. He also reported partially complying with commands to throw things by picking up an object but not throwing it. Furthermore, he said that he complied with commands to 'wash your hands' 50 per cent of the time because he believed that something harmful might happen to him or his mother, or someone might die, if he resisted.

According to Kevin, the voices often decreased after compliance but sometimes laughed at him. If he resisted, the voices got louder and made him feel more scared. Pre-therapy, Kevin reported that he was 70 per cent convinced that he would act on serious commands to harm himself or others.

At the time of the assessment, Kevin was rated as at 'high risk of acting on the voices' commands, with likely harm to self and others', and was rated as 'reporting high levels of distress associated with the commands'.

Beliefs about identity and meaning

Kevin was 80 per cent convinced that he heard voices because he had been bullied at school. Moreover, he believed that the female voice sounded like his mother because of its accent, although he had no idea why he heard this particular voice.

Target behaviours

The main compliance behaviours targeted for intervention were acting on commands to harm himself or others, and commands to wash his hands.

Stage 2: Intervention stage

Presentation and engagement in therapy

Kevin presented as a timid, rather immature and lonely young man: he reported having few friends of his own age, mostly relying on his mother and her partner for social opportunities.

In the first session, the therapist met with Kevin initially, and obtained his permission to meet with his mother and her partner at the end of the session in order to explain the aims of therapy and to answer any questions. It was emphasised that Kevin would be encouraged to take increasing responsibility for managing his difficulties, with support from the therapist. By the end of the session, Kevin appeared enthusiastic to participate and his carers seemed happy to encourage his attendance on a weekly basis.

In session two, Kevin reported that the voices had criticised therapy, saying 'it will all go wrong', and 'it's hopeless seeing her, she can't do anything'. Initially, Kevin's response was to feel disappointed but he described feeling more hopeful than the voices. Further discussion revealed that Kevin often disagreed with the voices, even though they did not like it and he felt scared for standing up to them. The therapist praised Kevin for being honest with her and encouraged him to 'give therapy a go' despite the voices' negative responses.

Throughout the sessions Kevin remained well motivated to engage in therapy. He attended regularly, and was very keen to talk about his experiences and to complete homework tasks.

Challenging beliefs about control over the voices

Over the sessions, a number of coping strategies were identified that seemed to help alleviate Kevin's distress in association with the voices. Distraction techniques included talking with or being in the company of someone he trusts, reading a good book out loud (quietly), listening to relaxing music, playing computer games, drawing or painting, going out for a walk and generally keeping occupied.

For some voice hearers, focusing on the voices has been found to reduce voice frequency (Nelson, 1997). A technique was suggested that involved

Kevin choosing to focus on the voices at set times. Kevin would say something like 'I can't listen to you right now, come back at two o'clock and I'll listen then'. At the set time, Kevin would decide how to cope with the voices. For example, he could listen to the voices without responding, trying to remain as relaxed as possible, or he could shadow the voices, repeating word for word what was said, or he could challenge the voices by questioning what they said. Alternatively, he could choose to tell the voices to 'stop' or 'leave me alone' in a firm way.

In addition, it was observed that Kevin often felt very anxious when hearing the voices. Consequently, anxiety management strategies were encouraged, including the use of a relaxation tape, breathing exercises and problem solving.

As Kevin used coping strategies more frequently, he noticed that the voices began to quieten down.

Exploring beliefs around compliance with or resistance of command voices

Pre-therapy, Kevin believed that he had to comply with the voices' commands because he feared that the voices might harm him or someone he cared about if he resisted. This belief was challenged in therapy, as follows.

- It was proposed that only something physical, like a knife or a bullet, can harm the physical body. Gradually, Kevin began to develop the belief that the voices were not physical objects, thus concluding that they could not do him any physical harm.
- It was observed that the voices seemed to rely on Kevin to do what they said. The therapist explored what happened when Kevin chose *not* to act. Kevin began to realise that he had resisted the voices' commands many times without him or his family coming to any harm. He concluded that the voices could not physically make him comply and that they were powerless to act themselves.
- It was acknowledged that the words the voices used, their loud volume and their aggressive tone often scared Kevin. Nonetheless, it was emphasised that words alone could not *physically* harm him.
- Furthermore, Kevin had previously believed that he must obey the voices because they said things again and again. Kevin observed that the voices tended to repeat themselves often (for example, repeatedly telling him to wash his hands). It was suggested that these sounds may have been fragments of memory that were stuck, like a broken record, in part of his brain so that they kept coming round and round.

Kevin concluded that just because the voices say things repeatedly in an aggressive, loud way, this does not make them true or right, and does not mean that he has to agree with them. Moreover, just because the voices tell Kevin to do something, this does not mean he has to do it or that they have the power to make him act: he can choose whether or not to comply.

Through Socratic dialogue, the advantages and disadvantages of acting on commands were explored, particularly those commands with serious consequences for himself or others. Disadvantages of obeying included harming himself or others, the risk of getting into trouble with the police and feeling very distressed. In addition, Kevin observed that the voices sometimes continued even after he had complied, and when they did stop it was only for a short time as they would return the next time he was anxious or angry about something.

Advantages of resisting included no risk of getting into trouble or putting himself in danger, feeling more in control because he had chosen not to act and no physical harm coming to Kevin or significant others. It was noted that while Kevin often felt anxious at first, when resisting the voices' commands, this anxiety did gradually reduce, especially when he distracted himself in some way or tried breathing and relaxation exercises. He concluded that there were more advantages to resisting the voices' commands than complying with them.

Gradually, Kevin became less fearful that the voices could harm him if he resisted their commands. Consequently, he felt more able to choose when he complied or resisted. For example, he decided that it was OK to wash his hands once after going to the toilet or getting them dirty but no more than that, but he decided that he would resist any commands to harm himself or other people, or to throw things. Kevin came to the conclusion that the voices were not as powerful as he had previously thought, and that he was more powerful than he used to believe: he began to consider his relationship with the voices as more equal.

Exploring beliefs about the power and control of the voice

By trying the various different coping strategies described earlier, Kevin began to believe that he had more control over the voices. This was used as evidence to support an emerging belief that he had as much power as the voices.

Challenging beliefs that the voices could make Kevin harm himself or others gave further support for the view that the voices were not as powerful as he had previously thought, and that he was more powerful than he used to believe.

Kevin began to believe that he had more control because he could decide whether or not to agree with or believe what the voices said, and he could choose whether or not to act on what they said.

At the beginning of therapy, Kevin suggested that the voices might have caused his grandmother's death: he had believed that the voices had told her to smoke lots of cigarettes, which might have caused her to develop cancer. In therapy this belief was challenged in order to reduce the level of power Kevin was attributing to the voices by holding them responsible for his grand-mother's death. With great care and sensitivity, Socratic questioning was used to explore the possibility that his grandmother had chosen to smoke cigarettes but may not have been aware of the risks to her physical health. By the end of therapy, Kevin was convinced that the death of his grandmother was not caused by the voices.

Near the end of therapy, Kevin reported acting on the voices' commands to climb out of his bedroom window late at night. He said that he was then caught by local police breaking into a building and was given a verbal warning. The event was explored, including the advantages and disadvantages of acting on the commands, and possible alternatives to acting. Kevin's responsibility for choosing whether or not to act was emphasised. It was hypothesised that Kevin's behaviour could have been partly explained as an attempt to be a rebellious young adult and assert his independence.

Exploring beliefs about identity

During therapy, Kevin reported that he heard the voices of bullies from his old school. The therapist proposed a possible alternative explanation for these experiences, namely as *memories* of the voices of those bullies from the past. It was explained that the part of Kevin's brain that recognises different people's voices might be automatically but wrongly activated at stressful times, causing Kevin to hear voices that *sound like* the bullies. According to Nelson (1997: 187), voices that are more familiar or voices that are of particular importance to the person are more likely to be wrongly activated. In Kevin's case, it was suggested that whenever he was feeling upset or angry he would be reminded of the bullies, which was likely to trigger those particular voices inside his head.

In addition, images of the bullies that seemed very real to Kevin were sometimes triggered at stressful times. As a consequence, Kevin believed that some of the bullies continued to live nearby. He was asked to describe the images in detail: he recalled that the boys in the images were 13 or 14 years old, wore school uniform and they looked exactly as they had looked when Kevin was at secondary school. However, it was observed that today they would be 18 or 19 years old and, most likely, dressed differently. This was used as evidence to suggest that the images were vivid *memories* of the bullies from the past, rather than actual people in the present.

Furthermore, Kevin reported having images of the bullies punching and kicking him, on occasions, as if it was happening in the present moment. However, there was never any evidence of fresh bruises afterwards, suggesting that Kevin was reliving unpleasant events from the past. Gradually, Kevin became increasingly convinced that the voices and images of the bullies were memories from the past rather than real people in the here and now.

Pre-therapy, Kevin had believed that the female voice sounded somewhat like his mother. Again, erroneous activation of the voice recognition centre in the brain was proposed to explain this.

Exploring beliefs about meaning

Pre-therapy, Kevin believed that the voices were somehow related to the bullies from his old school. The stress/vulnerability model was introduced as a way of explaining why Kevin's mental health difficulties, including hearing voices and extreme anxiety, might have developed. This model suggests that people may have a greater or lesser predisposition to psychotic experiences or other physical/mental health symptoms, which are triggered by higher or lower numbers of stressful events experienced.

A number of factors were identified that might have contributed to the development of Kevin's mental health problems, including witnessing his father's anger at a young age; the absence of a male role model from the age of three years; part self-blame for his father leaving the family home; finding reading and writing difficult at school; being regularly bullied over a period of four years at senior school, leading to post-traumatic memories of events; and coping with the loss of significant others, i.e. his absent father and the recent death of his grandmother.

It was concluded that Kevin heard distressing voices as a result of a build-up of stresses in his life. His current ability to cope better with his difficulties and to build on his strengths, with the help and support of others, was emphasised.

Other issues addressed in the therapy

Bereavement

During therapy it became clear that Kevin was still trying to come to terms with the recent loss of his grandmother. He recalled how he had been mentally unwell when she became ill and subsequently died, and he had been unable to attend her funeral. Also, he had not visited her grave, which was located some distance away from where he lived. Kevin agreed to write his grandmother a goodbye letter: he later reported that he had enjoyed writing it despite crying. Kevin was encouraged to express his feelings around her death and to remember the good times they had spent together.

Relationship with his father

The issue of Kevin's father leaving when he was young was explored. As a child, Kevin had blamed himself for his father's departure and failure to visit subsequently; as a young adult, he was able to consider alternative explanations that attributed responsibility to his parents. Kevin described feeling sad and angry that his father had been absent for most of his childhood. It was hypothesised that Kevin's tendency to throw things when angry might have been a learned behaviour from his father.

Sexuality

Kevin reported that he was unsure about his sexual orientation, although further discussion revealed that his knowledge of homosexuality seemed limited and somewhat naive. Some basic education around these issues was offered, with emphasis on sexuality being a personal choice and the importance of both adults consenting to sex within a sexual relationship.

Bullying

Bullying was a common theme throughout Kevin's childhood and young adulthood (indeed, Kevin had attributed the identity of some of the voices to the bullies at school). Kevin described how he had only had a few friends at school as he was generally mistrustful of people. He had tried to defend himself against the bullies but had found it difficult to stand up for himself. More recently, Kevin reported having to cope with neighbours' children throwing stones at him. In therapy, ways of being more assertive were explored and recommendations were made for further assertiveness training once therapy ended.

Anger management

Kevin revealed that he sometimes acted on command voices when he was frustrated with something or someone. For example, he described how he had thrown a vase in response to the voices' command after being unable to fix his radio. Alternative ways of releasing frustration without damaging objects or hitting people were explored, and the fact that Kevin could have chosen not to act was discussed. Increased arousal levels were linked with the voices being triggered.

Hand-washing behaviour

Although Kevin reported that the voices frequently commanded him to wash his hands, discussion revealed that hand-washing often functioned to alleviate feelings of anxiety or anger: 'it's as if I am trying to wash my problems away'. Kevin came to the conclusion that washing his hands did not really make him feel any better. Consequently, more adaptive ways of managing anxiety and anger were explored:

- Talking to someone he trusts, telling them how he is feeling.
- Using breathing and relaxation exercises.
- Lifting his mood by doing something enjoyable or something he gains a sense of achievement from; for example, drawing or painting, chatting to someone or attending college.
- Being more assertive – expressing his feelings in a clear, calm way (rather than shouting or throwing things).
- Expressing his anger in a positive way (e.g. writing his feelings down in a private notebook).

Sleeping difficulties

From the outset of therapy, Kevin reported having occasional problems in getting to sleep or in waking up in the night, particularly when he was worried about something. Alternatives strategies to pacing up and down were discussed, including distraction techniques (such as listening to music on a personal stereo or reading a good book) or writing down concerns and a plan of action, then planning to deal with it the next day.

Worrying and problem solving

It was identified that worrying about things often made Kevin feel anxious and depressed, as well as resulting in the voices becoming louder and more frequent. The concept of problem solving was introduced: first, the problem that was worrying Kevin needed to be identified; next, he was encouraged to consider whether the worry was realistic or exaggerated by asking himself 'what's the evidence for this worry?' Then he was encouraged to generate different solutions (seeking advice or support from others if necessary), and to choose the best solution. Finally, he needed to plan how to carry it out.

For example, he was worried about taking a taxi to college for fear of being mugged, beaten or stabbed by the taxi driver. Through talking with the therapist, he identified that it was very unlikely that this could happen, because: he had been in taxis before and nothing like this had happened; he did not know of this happening to anyone that he knew; and he could always check the taxi driver's ID and make sure that he was licensed. The evidence suggested that he was likely to be safe travelling to college in a taxi (with a licensed taxi driver).

In another example, he identified that he was worried about being bullied at college. He decided to speak to an education adviser, who suggested that he apply for a place at a special needs school where he would feel safer and better supported. This is what he did.

Balanced lifestyle

Education around a healthy, balanced lifestyle was introduced with a view to minimising the impact of current stressors on Kevin's mental health. Strategies included knowing his own limits (i.e. keeping busy but not over-doing it to the point of feeling anxious or irritable); keeping active as a distraction from the voices as well as reducing boredom; taking things one step at a time, with breaks in between; recognising that a setback was also a learning opportunity; having a good amount of sleep and eating well. Kevin's own resources for coping with stress were emphasised, in addition to seeking help and support from others, and maintaining a good support network.

Outcome

By the end of therapy, Kevin reported that he was hearing the voices less frequently and that the majority of the voices were distressing to a moderate degree (compared to very distressing pre-therapy). He believed that he was able to have some control over the voices on the majority of occasions. Fur-thermore, he believed that he was much more powerful than and much stronger than the voices, much superior to them, and somewhat more con-fident and somewhat more knowledgeable than the voices. He no longer believed that the voices could physically harm him.

Kevin reported that he chose to resist commands to wash his hands on the majority of occasions (about 70 per cent of the time) by using a variety of coping strategies. Moreover, he was convinced that he would not act on commands to harm himself or others because of the serious consequences.

Significant changes in beliefs about the identity and meaning of the voices were reported by the end of therapy. Kevin no longer believed that the voices were the actual bullies from his old school; instead he believed that the voices, which *sounded like* these bullies, were mistakenly generated by his brain, particularly at times of stress. Furthermore, he believed the voices had developed as a result of a build-up of stresses in his life.

Pre-therapy and post-therapy measures for Kevin are summarised in Table 10.1. The Voice Power Differential Scale (VPDS; Birchwood *et al.*, 2000; Appendix 1, this volume) and the control and distress scales of the Psychotic Symptom Rating Scales (PSYRATS; Haddock *et al.*, 1999) were adminis-tered before and after the intervention. The VPDS measures the power differ-ential between voice and voice hearer on five-point scales, with regard to overall power and a number of related characteristics. The PSYRATS meas-ures the severity of a number of dimensions of auditory hallucinations and

Table 10.1 Summary comparing pre- and post-therapy measures for Kevin

Measure		Pre-therapy	Post-therapy (6-month follow-up)	Post-therapy (12-month follow-up)
Power differential[1]	Power	4	2	3
	Strength	5	2	1
	Confidence	4	1	1
	Knowledge	3	3	5
	Harm	5	3	1
	Superior	1	1	1
Control over the voices[2]		4	1	2
Distress[2]		3	4	2

[1] Voice Power Differential Scale (VPDS).
[2] Psychotic Symptom Rating Scale (PSYRATS).

delusions, including amount and intensity of distress associated with these symptoms.

The results in Table 10.1 indicate significant positive changes in Kevin's beliefs about the power and control of the voices by the end of therapy and at 12-month follow-up. Post-therapy, he believed that he was more powerful, stronger and much more confident than the voices, and much superior to the voices; he also believed that he and they had about the same amount of knowledge and were equally able to harm each other. At 12-month follow-up, Kevin rated himself as much stronger and much more confident than the voices, superior to them, and more able to harm them than they were able to harm him, although he rated that he and the voices had about the same amount of power. Furthermore, there was a significant improvement in Kevin's beliefs about control over the voices: post-therapy he believed that he could have some control over the voices on the majority of occasions. At 12-month follow-up, he believed that he could have some control over the voices approximately half the time. Finally, Kevin rated the voices as extremely distressing post-therapy, but this had reduced to moderately distressing at 12-month follow-up.

Conclusion

Kevin reported that he had enjoyed the therapy sessions and had found them helpful. In the therapist's view, he had benefited from talking about the voices and other issues, and learning adaptive strategies for coping with the voices, as well as managing symptoms of anxiety and anger.

Recommendations

At the end of therapy, the following recommendations were made by the therapist, for support staff to pursue.

- Regular support sessions with a keyworker to review the work achieved in therapy, and to enable Kevin to discuss relevant issues, such as sexuality, loss and relationships with peers and adults.
- With regard to sexuality, it was hypothesised that Kevin could be vulnerable to abuse by others. Further education around assertiveness, individual rights and sexual preferences was recommended.
- Discussion around managing relationships with his peers was recommended to minimise the likelihood of further bullying, particularly at college.
- Family work with Kevin's mother and her partner was also suggested. Firstly, there was concern that some of Kevin's behaviours were being mistakenly attributed to his mental health problems or biological causes, rather than being seen in light of 'normal' rebellious adolescent behaviour. Secondly, dependency issues could be explored; for example, enabling Kevin to become a more independent young adult.
- To use the summary handout provided by the therapist to regularly review their work together, with particular emphasis on Kevin's ability to stand up to the voices and to get on with his life in spite of them (for example, encouraging Kevin to continue attending college).

Chapter 11

Does CBT for CH work?

Findings from a randomised controlled trial

We hope that the previous chapters have given the reader/practitioner a good grounding in the theory and practice of cognitive therapy for command hallucinations, and have conveyed an impression of its overall reasonable effectiveness, on the basis of the outcomes, for most of the cases we have described.

However, the evidence of positive change on the basis of 'before' and 'after' measures for a number of cases is not sufficient for a valid demonstration of its effectiveness. Effectiveness can only be shown by means of proper, scientific outcome studies – either single-case experimental design studies or randomised controlled trials. The evidence from such studies for CBT for psychosis in general is reasonably encouraging. As we discussed in Chapter 2, meta-analyses of trials that met required standards of scientific rigour (Cormac et al., 2002; Pilling et al., 2002) found that CBT in addition to standard care (relative to standard care alone) has a beneficial effect regarding the positive symptoms. However, none of the trials focused on command hallucinations and their outcomes were traditional scores on psychosis scales (e.g. Positive and Negative Syndrome Scale (PANSS)) rather than on compliance/behaviour and distress. In Chapter 2 we asserted that treating CBT as a 'quasi-neuroleptic' in this way was an anomaly, and would not produce the most effective therapy or research precision in detecting change in the most important variables, namely distress and dysfunctional behaviour. We therefore undertook a randomised controlled trial of the type we recommend, to test the efficacy of CBT for CH on distress and compliance or appeasement, thereby testing with precision whether the theory is supported. The eight cases described above were participants in the trial. In this chapter we describe this trial – how we recruited, engaged and assessed the participants, the method we used to carry out the evaluation, the results of the evaluation and the implications of the results, and indeed of the development of this alternative-to-medication, or at least adjunct-to-medication, approach to a problem hitherto presumed intractable. A more detailed account of the trial is available (Trower et al., 2004).

The aims of the trial

With the support of a Department of Health grant we carried out a single-blind, intention-to-treat randomised controlled trial in which we compared the efficacy of CBT for CH versus treatment as usual (TAU) in a sample of participants with command hallucinations considered at high risk of further compliance by virtue of their recent history. The purpose of the trial was to evaluate whether CBT for CH could, by targeting power beliefs, reduce compliance and/or appeasement and distress, and increase resistance. The main hypothesis and primary outcome was that the CBT for CH group compared to the control group would show a lower level of compliance and appeasement behaviour and an increase in resistance. The secondary outcomes were: (1) a lower conviction in the power and social rank superiority of voices and in the need to comply, (2) a reduction in distress and depression. No changes in the topography of voices (frequency, loudness, content) were predicted since our intervention was aimed at the beliefs and not the symptoms, and if we reduced or eradicated compliance and distress, we would consider that a successful outcome.

Method

The participants were recruited from local mental health services in Birmingham and Solihull, Sandwell and a West Midlands semi-secure unit for mentally ill offenders. Inclusion criteria were that patients conform to an ICD10 diagnosis of schizophrenia or related disorder with command hallucinations for at least six months. Participants were required to have a recent history of compliance with and appeasement of voices with 'severe' commands, including harm to self or others or major social transgressions. Patients were excluded where there was a primary organic or addictive disorder.

All aspects of recruitment, screening and outcome assessment were organised and administered by an experienced research associate, Mrs Angela Nelson, over a two-year period between September 2000 and July 2002. All referrals were offered an interview to establish eligibility and to obtain consent, and there was a further interview for eligible patients for assessment in terms of the outcome measures (see below). (Because of the importance of effective and standardised recruitment, screening and assessment, the whole procedure was manualised; it is given in Appendix 2.) Eligible and consenting patients were then randomly assigned to TAU or CBT for CH-plus-TAU for a period of six months. Participants were post-tested at six months after CBT for CH or TAU and again at 12-month follow-ups.

Measures of cognitions and behaviours, symptoms and affect relevant to the hypotheses were given at pre-test, post-test and follow-up. The main measures were the same as those described in Chapter 2, and included the Cognitive Assessment Schedule (CAS), Beliefs about Voices Questionnaire

(BAVQ), Voice Power Differential Scale (VPDS), Omniscience Scale (OS), Positive and Negative Syndrome Scale (PANSS), Psychotic Symptom Rating Scales (PSYRATS) and the Calgary Depression Scale for Schizophrenia (CDSS). We also used the Voice Compliance Scale (VCS) which, as pointed out in Chapter 2, is an observer-rated scale to measure the frequency of CH and level of compliance/resistance with each identified command. The VCS was completed in two stages. Firstly, the trial assessor, Angela Nelson, using a structured interview format, obtained from each client a description of all those commands and associated behaviours (compliance or resistance) within the previous eight weeks where they felt compelled to respond. She then interviewed either a keyworker or relative to corroborate the information, and, where there was a discrepancy, recorded the worst behaviour mentioned by either party. Secondly, she classified each behaviour as: neither appease-ment nor compliant (1); symbolic appeasement, i.e. compliant with innocu-ous and/or harmless commands (2); appeasement, i.e. preparatory acts or gestures (3); partial compliance with at least one severe command (4), full compliance with at least one severe command (5). The behaviours were also independently and blindly rated using the information collated from the informants by three of the authors, and were found to have good reliability.

The findings

Sixty-nine individuals were identified as being eligible for the study and were invited to participate. Of these, 31 refused consent, leaving a sample of 38 consenting to randomisation. The sample included 24 males and 14 females, with a mean age of 35.5 years (SD: 10.4). The sample was drawn from a broad ethnic base, including 27 (71 per cent) white, 6 (16 per cent) Black Caribbean, and 4 (11 per cent) other (South Asian).

All patients reported two or more commands from the 'dominant' voice, at least one of which was a 'severe' command. The most severe commands were to kill self (25), kill others (13), harm self (12) and harm others (14). Less severe commands involved innocuous, day-to-day behaviour (wash dishes, masturbate, take a bath) and minor social transgressions (e.g. break windows, shout out loud, swear in public).

Participants were considered at high risk of compliance since 30 (79 per cent) had complied, 14 (37 per cent) had appeased and 29 (76 per cent) had expressed the fear that the voices would either harm or kill them or a family member if they did not comply. The compliance rate is at the high end of the range for recent studies (Shawyer et al., 2003) because our sampling strategy involved identifying those considered to have recently complied.

Five participants in the sample had been prosecuted or cautioned for behaviour linked to voices' commands. This included causing actual bodily harm on a minor, grievous bodily harm, theft and common assault. Three participants had been hospitalised (two detained under the Mental Health

Act, 1983) for attempting to kill someone in response to voices within the previous three years.

A further indication of the severity of need in this sample was the heavy and prolonged consumption of TAU, both during the trial and as sampled one year prior to the trial. TAU involved 19 categories of services and admissions, as shown in Table 11.1. Another indication of severity was the fact that at the time of consent to enter the trial, eight were hospitalised, two being admitted under Section 3 and one under Section 2 of the Mental Health Act (1983), and another five being informal admissions.

The treatment group completed a median of 16 sessions. Five participants (27 per cent) in the treatment group dropped out prematurely, attending between 4 and 12 sessions. This drop-out rate is comparable to other trials of

Table 11.1 Service consumption and treatment as usual during the trial and one year prior to the trial

	Year prior to trial		During trial	
	TAU	CTCH	TAU	CTCH
Services				
Outpatients	85%	89%	100%	89%
CPN	50%	33%	60%	56%
Day centre	45%	38%	35%	28%
Social worker	0%	22%	25%	11%
Supported accommodation	30%	22%	55%	28%
Support worker	25%	50%	45%	11%
Community drug team	5%	6%	5%	0%
Probation officer	5%	6%	5%	6%
Occupational therapist	35%	22%	20%	11%
Psychologist	15%*	16%*	5%†	6%†
Respite care	0%	6%	5%	6%
Home treatment team	22%	6%	20%	6%
Art therapy	10%	6%	5%	0%
Voices group	0%	6%	0%	0%
Admissions				
Informal	20%	22%	15%	22%
Section 2	10%	0%	5%	6%
Section 3	15%	0%	15%	0%
ECT	0%	0%	0%	6%
Guardianship order	0%	6%	0%	6%

TAU, treatment as usual; CTCH, cognitive therapy for command hallucinations plus treatment as usual.
* Psychological input in the treatment group included anger management, childhood trauma and symptom management. Psychological input in the control group constituted anxiety and anger management.
† Psychological input for the treatment group constituted anger management. Psychological input in the control group constituted anxiety management.

this type. The intention was to include all 18 CBT participants at follow-up (including the drop-outs) but at six months three participants were lost to follow-up through withdrawal of consent, and a further one was lost at 12 months. In the control group two were lost to follow-up at six months (both died, one to natural causes and one to suicide), and two were lost at 12 months. There was no difference between groups in number lost to follow-up.

The impact of CBT for CH

How did they do? From 100 per cent compliance (the selection criterion) they all dropped significantly, the TAU to 53 per cent but the CBT group significantly more: over 12 months to only 14 per cent still complying or appeasing. If this very large reduction was due specifically to cognitive therapy we would also expect to see a change in conviction in the power beliefs. In fact that is what we did find. The CBT group reported a large and significant reduction in their beliefs in the power of the dominant voice, compared to TAU, which showed no change; this effect of CBT was maintained at 12-month follow-up. Furthermore, when we statistically removed the effect of the power beliefs, the treatment effect disappeared, providing further evidence that belief change was responsible for the reduction in compliance.

The belief in voices' omniscience also fell significantly in the CBT group but not in the TAU group, and this pattern was also maintained at 12 months. However, there was no impact of CBT on the perceived malevolence of voices at 6 months or 12 months. Patients receiving CBT also showed a significant improvement in perceived control over voices, compared to TAU, which showed no change. This pattern was maintained at 12 months.

Turning to the effect of CBT on distress and depression, we found that the intensity of distress fell significantly in the CBT group at 6 months but not in the control group. By 12 months, distress in the groups was no longer different but there was an overall lessening of distress over this period. By 12 months, depression had risen significantly in TAU but not in the CBT group.

Findings for voice topography were largely in line with predictions. Perceived voice frequency fell in the CBT group compared to TAU, which did not change from baseline. This difference was not maintained at 12 months. Voice loudness did not change in either group, nor did the reported negative content of voices.

Although we had no hypotheses about change in psychotic symptoms, there was in fact a significant drop in PANSS positive symptoms in the CBT group, and a small increase in the control group. Similarly, there was a small but consistent reduction in negative symptoms and general psychopathology in the CTCH group. These effects were maintained at 12 months for positive and negative symptoms and general psychopathology.

Within the PANSS positive scale, however, hallucinations showed no change at 6 months, or 12 months, in line with our expectations. For the delusions subscale, on the other hand, there was a reduction in the CBT group at 6 months, sustained at 12 months. Within the general psycho-pathology scale, there were significant changes in anxiety at 6 and 12 months, in tension at 6 months and in guilty thinking at 6 months.

Within the negative symptoms scale, there was a significant reduction in attention/concentration at 6 months and disturbance of volition at 6 months and 12 months.

There was no correlation between neuroleptic dose and PANSS positive symptoms at any point.

We have argued (from social rank theory) that compliance with a powerful dominant (voice) will vary as a function of (a) the power differential between the dominant (voice) and subordinate (voice hearer), (b) the distress or fear experienced and (c) beliefs about non-compliance (see Gilbert, 1992). A cor-relation matrix at 6 months showed that voice compliance was significantly correlated with both greater distress and power, thus supporting this aspect of our theory.

Implications

It is important to reiterate that the people in this study were selected as being at 'high risk': they had complied with 'serious' commands to self-harm, harm others or commit major social transgressions; they were highly distressed; and many were 'appeasing' the dominant voice in order to 'buy time' to avoid what they believed to be catastrophic consequences. Many had a history of forensic involvement, all were supported by community teams who referred the patients because of perceived risk and the clinicians involved acknowledged equipoise in their management.

The data presented here suggests that CBT for CH, in the context of good quality and a high level of TAU services, exerts a major influence on the risk of compliance, reduces distress and prevents the escalation of depression, compared to TAU alone. Depression is known to be high in this group from previous research (Birchwood *et al.*, 2000), confirmed in this study. Because of the selection criterion of recent compliance, it was likely that compliance behaviour would reduce over the 6- and 12-month periods ('regression to the mean'); however, given the high-risk status of this group, we may expect an increasing number of people complying with commands as further time elapses. Nevertheless, the 12-month clinical impact of CBT was significant. Perhaps more importantly, the risk factors for compliance in the CBT group had reduced markedly, particularly the perceived power of the voice, its omniscience and controllability, and the need to appease (14 per cent of the CBT group were appeasing or complying vs 53 per cent of TAU).

In line with our prediction, neither the topography nor the negative content of voices shifted (according to the self-reports of participants on the PSYR-ATS), with the exception of a temporary reduction in perceived frequency during the first 6 months. This underlines our view (Birchwood and Spencer, 2002) that CBT is most effective with beliefs (delusional or otherwise), rather than the primary psychotic experience, in this case auditory hallucinations. The focus of CBT is to change fundamentally the nature of the individual's relationship with his voices by challenging the power and omnipotence of his voices, thus reducing the motivation to comply. We concede, however, that if these treatment gains are sustained, the reduction of distress might well exert a beneficial influence on the frequency of voices. In a similar vein, we previously observed the similarity between the nature and content of voices and negative thoughts in depression (Gilbert *et al.*, 2001); relieving depression in this sample may likewise act to reduce the frequency and negative content of voices, though in the timescale observed here, only limited change was noted.

The reduction in PANSS positive symptoms was modest but consistent in the CBT group, leading to a highly significant and sustained effect. The hallucinations subscale showed a non-significant decline over 6 months, which disappeared at 12 months, once more underlining our contention that voice activity *per se* is not affected. PANSS delusions, on the other hand, showed a significant reduction at 6 and 12 months. This may well reflect the observed changes in the perceived power of the persecutor, in this instance the voice. PANSS general psychopathology showed the largest and most sustained reduction, particularly in social avoidance, attention and concentration.

Our primary dependent measure – compliance with commands – is not a straightforward concept (Beck-Sander *et al.*, 1997), as compliance can include covert as well as overt acts, and patients may also appease their voices by complying with less serious commands (a 'safety behaviour'). Our measure, developed from our earlier work (Beck-Sander *et al.*, 1997), recognises these subtleties and requires evidence from the client, but also from his relatives or case manager. The rating of this scale was undertaken by three raters in the first instance to establish inter-rater reliability.

We are encouraged that the study also found (predicted) changes in power, distress/depression and omniscience (which were largely measured by self-report scales) and that these correlated significantly with our primary outcome, compliance; indeed, when power was controlled for, the effect on compliance was rendered non-significant. This adds strength to our claims that: (1) compliance was genuinely changed and the treatment effect was mediated by reduction in voice power, (2) CBT had broad effects on outcomes, but (3) the absence of (self-reported) change in voice activity argues against the notion that patients' ratings were unreliable, and measures simply reflected the operation of a 'halo' effect in favour of CBT across all measures.

Data obtained on prescription of neuroleptic and other drugs and provision of general mental health services during the course of the trial showed no difference between the groups and did not account for the effect of CBT, but did underline their high level of service use linked to perceived risk. This suggests that the impact of CBT we report here is unlikely to be accounted for by factors extraneous to the treatment. The pattern of neuroleptic use during the course of the trial showed no difference between the groups but did show a steady rise in neuroleptic prescription in the TAU group and a small *reduction* in the CBT group. This suggests that concern about risk led to a raising of the dose in those not receiving CBT; this may reflect concern in clinicians as much as perceived benefit from CBT.

The rise in neuroleptic use in TAU was correlated with reducing compliance; in CBT the opposite was observed, i.e. reducing compliance was in line with *reducing* medication. There is a theoretical possibility that TAU participants were under-medicated and that the rise in medication prescription was responsible for the reduction in compliance (this could not account for the reduction in compliance in CBT). This strikes us as unlikely for three reasons. Firstly, both groups were receiving medication well in excess of BNF (British Medical Association and Royal Pharmaceutical Society of Great Britain, 2001) and other guidelines, including widespread use of atypicals, and Clozapine; second, at no point did dose correlate with compliance, power or PANSS scores; third, using drug dose as covariate did not affect the results. If TAU were under-medicated, this would serve to underestimate the effect size of CBT as compliance would be less likely to change over time. We believe that these differential changes in medication prescription reflect, as we indicate above, (understandable) clinician anxiety about this very high-risk group.

Nevertheless, it remains a possibility that non-specific aspects of the therapy were responsible for the effects. We believe, however, that the large correlation between changes in voice power and compliance by six months (0.63) strongly supports our contention that this aspect of the relationship with the voice (power) is the key independent variable. Whether CBT alone brought about this change cannot be determined from these data, though we have clear evidence that the therapist adhered to protocol and therefore we can be reasonably confident that the intervention itself was targeted at voice power and compliance.

The 'real world' relevance of the study, we feel, is particularly strong. The sample as a whole was a severely distressed and generally a high-risk group. Approximately 55 per cent of those eligible took part (i.e. 38 out of 69), and 27 per cent dropped out of the CBT group, which is average for CBT in this population (Norman and Townsend, 1999; Durham *et al.*, 2003). Given that this was a high-risk group, we looked at the reasons for drop-out, and found for example that one person believed that the voice might harm or kill them for disclosing too much information; another feared that talking during therapy made the voices worse and continued on condition that she could determine how much she disclosed about the voices.

The client group in this study – all experiencing command hallucinations and all having recently acted upon their commands – is typical of one of the highest risk groups in psychiatry, who represent a major concern to their case managers, responsible medical officers (RMOs), relatives, but particularly themselves. This group is generally regarded as treatment resistant, including medication or CBT ('conventional' CBT for psychosis is less effective with voices (Birchwood and Spencer, 2002) and the clinicians involved acknowledge equipoise in their management, as witnessed by the high level of referral to the trial). Our study – and the cases described in detail in Chapters 4 to 10 – showed that many clients felt themselves caught helplessly in a vortex of voice power, but found that CBT for CH gave them an opportunity to exert control by distancing themselves from their assumption about voice power. For example, one client commented that 'I know now that the voices can't hurt me – I feel that I am in control now. I still hear the voices but they are not as powerful.' Another client directly attributed his improvement to using 'all the techniques that she [SB] taught me and not only have the voices disappeared but I am sleeping and eating properly now'. CBT for CH is therefore responding to a major gap in the treatment for people with ongoing distressing voices, and deserves further evaluation.

This study was not definitive. It has suggested an effect size of major clinical significance, but because the sample size was small and the study was conducted in only one part of the country, there is a need to replicate the study in a large-scale randomised controlled trial incorporating different loci and different therapists, affording the opportunity to understand for whom CBT is most effective and how durable any effects may be. The durability question is of particular importance. There is a strand of psychiatric opinion that treatments for schizophrenia are effective only as long as they are active (McGlashan, 1988); perhaps, therefore, a more theoretical and clinically relevant question might be 'how much further intervention is required to *maintain* the effect of treatment?' We are currently developing a multi-centre study to test CBT for CH in a large sample from various centres in the UK.

Epilogue

In this book we have attempted to present an innovative approach to therapy with this most difficult and refractory of client groups. A thread running through our approach has been the integration of cognitive theory, the results of over a decade of research onto the 'cognitive model' of voices informing what we believe to be a coherent intervention. We bring to this enterprise a firm belief that cognitive models and cognitive behaviour therapy should maintain their lineage in emotional dysfunction and focus on relieving distress and troublesome behaviour associated with psychosis symptoms and the psychosis diagnosis. What perhaps marks this as distinctive is the absence of the PANSS (Kay *et al.*, 1987), i.e. symptoms themselves as the primary outcome. For us the key to further research in this area is to understand the way in which anomalous interpersonal schemas affect the relationship with the dominant voice; to identify the developmental risk factors and trajectories that govern their development; and to explore the impact of intervening directly and exclusively with such schemas, including the exciting possibilities this offers for the primary prevention of distress and patienthood. We hope we have excited the reader sufficiently to share our passion for this prospectus.

References

Addington, D., Addington, J. and Maticka-Tyndale, E. (1993). Assessing depression in schizophrenia: the Calgary Depression Scale. *British Journal of Psychiatry*, *163* (suppl. 22), 39–44.

American Psychiatric Association (1994) *Diagnostic and statistical manual IV*. Washington, DC: APA.

Appelbaum, P.S., Robbins, P. and Monahan, J. (2000). Violence and delusions: data from the MacArthur Violence Risk Assessment. *American Journal of Psychiatry*, *157*, 566–572.

Beck, A.T. (1952). Successful outpatient psychotherapy of a chronic schizophrenic with a delusion based on borrowed guilt. *Psychiatry*, *15*, 305–312.

Beck, A.T., Rush, A.J., Shaw, B.F. and Emery, G. (1979). *Cognitive therapy of depression*. New York: Guilford.

Beck-Sander, A., Birchwood, M. and Chadwick, P. (1997). Acting on command hallucinations: a cognitive approach. *British Journal of Clinical Psychology*, *36*, 139–148.

Benjamin, L.S. (1989). Is chronicity a function of the relationship between the person and the auditory hallucination? *Schizophrenia Bulletin*, *15*, 291–310.

Birchwood, M. and Chadwick, P. (1997). The omnipotence of voices: testing the validity of a cognitive model. *Psychological Medicine*, *27*, 1345–1353.

Birchwood, M., Gilbert, P., Gilbert, J., Trower, P., Meaden, A., Murray, E. and Miles, J. (2004). Interpersonal and role-related schema influence the relationship with the dominant 'voice' in schizophrenia: a comparison of three models. *Psychological Medicine*, *34*, 1571–1580.

Birchwood, M., Meaden, A., Trower, P., Gilbert, P. and Plaistow, J. (2000). The power and omnipotence of voices: subordination and entrapment by voices and significant others. *Psychological Medicine*, *30*, 337–344.

Birchwood, M. and Spencer, E. (1999). Psychotherapies for schizophrenia. In M. Maj and N. Sartorius (Eds), *Schizophrenia. WPA series in evidence based psychiatry*. Chichester, UK: Wiley.

Birchwood, M. and Spencer, E. (2002). Psychotherapies for schizophrenia. In M. Maj and N. Sartorius (Eds), *Schizophrenia: WPA series in evidence based psychiatry*, 2nd ed., pp. 147–241. Chichester, UK: Wiley.

Bleuler, E. (1924). *Textbook of Psychiatry*. New York: Macmillan.

Braham, L., Trower, P. and Birchwood, M. (2004). Acting on command hallucinations and dangerous behavior: a critique of the major findings in the last decade. *Clinical Psychology Review*, *24*, 529–555.

Brennan, P., Mednick, S. and Hodges, S. (2000). Major mental disorders and criminal violence in a Danish birth cohort. *Archives of General Psychiatry*, *57*, 494–500.

Brett-Jones, J., Garety, P. and Hemsley, D. (1987). Measuring delusional experiences: a method and its application. *British Journal of Clinical Psychology*, *26*, 257–265.

British Medical Association and Royal Pharmaceutical Society of Great Britain (2001). British National Formulary (No. 39). London: BMA, RPS.

Brown, G.W., Harris, T.O. and Hepworth, C. (1995). Loss, humiliation, and entrapment among women developing depression: a patient and non-patient comparison. *Psychological Medicine*, *25*, 7–21.

Buchanan, A. (1993). Acting on delusion: a review. *Psychological Medicine*, *23*, 123–134.

Byrne, S., Trower, P., Birchwood, M., Meaden, A. and Nelson, A. (2003). Command hallucinations: cognitive theory, therapy and research. *Journal of Cognitive Psychotherapy*, *17*, 67–84.

Chadwick, P. and Birchwood, M.J. (1994). The omnipotence of voices: a cognitive approach to auditory hallucinations. *British Journal of Psychiatry*, *164*, 190–201.

Chadwick, P. and Birchwood, M. (1995). The omnipotence of voices II: The beliefs about voices questionnaire. *British Journal of Psychiatry*, *166*, 773–776.

Chadwick, P., Birchwood, M. and Trower, P. (1996). *Cognitive therapy for delusions, voices and paranoia*. Chichester, UK: Wiley.

Chadwick, P., Lees, S. and Birchwood, M. (2000). The revised beliefs about voices questionnaire (BAVQ-R). *British Journal of Psychiatry*, *177*, 229–232.

Chadwick P.D.J. and Lowe, C.F. (1990). Measurement and modification of delusional beliefs. *Journal of Consulting and Clinical Psychology*, *58*, 225–232.

Champion, A. and Power, M.J. (1995). Social and cognitive approaches to depression: towards a new synthesis. *British Journal of Clinical Psychology*, *34*, 485–503.

Close, H. and Garety, P. (1998). Cognitive assessment of voices: further developments in understanding the emotional impact of voices. *British Journal of Clinical Psychology*, *37*, 173–188.

Cormac, I., Jones, C. and Campbell, C. (2002). Cognitive behaviour therapy for schizophrenia. *Cochrane Dbase System Review*, *1*, CD000524.

Drayton, M., Birchwood, M. and Trower, P. (1998). Early attachment experience and recovery from psychosis. *British Journal of Clinical Psychology*, *37*, 269–284.

Drury, V., Birchwood, M., Cochrane, R. and Macmillan, F. (1996). Cognitive therapy and recovery form acute psychosis: a controlled trial II. Impact on recovery time. *British Journal of Psychiatry*, *169*, 602–607.

Dryden, W. (1995). *Brief rational emotive behaviour therapy*. Chichester, UK: Wiley.

Durham, R.C., Guthrie, M., Morton, R.V., Reid, D.A., Treliving, L.R., Fowler, D. and Macdonald, R.R. (2003). Tayside-Fife clinical trial of cognitive behavioural therapy for medication-resistant psychotic symptoms. Results to 3-month follow-up. *British Journal of Psychiatry*, *182*, 303–311.

Fleiss, J. (1981). *Statistical methods for rates and proportions*. Chichester, UK: Wiley.

Fowler, D., Garety, P. and Kuipers, E. (1995). *Cognitive behaviour therapy for psychosis*. Chichester, UK: Wiley.

Gilbert, P. (1989). *Human nature and suffering*. Hove, UK: Lawrence Erlbaum Associates.

Gilbert, P. (1992). *Depression: the evolution of powerlessness*. Hove, UK: Lawrence Erlbaum Associates.

Gilbert, P., Birchwood, M., Gilbert, J., Trower, P., Hay, J., Murray, B., Meaden, A., Olsen, K. and Miles, J.N. (2001). An exploration of evolved mental mechanisms for dominant and subordinate behaviour in relation to auditory hallucinations in schizophrenia and critical thoughts in depression. *Psychological Medicine, 31*, 1117–1127.

Gould, R.A. Mueser, K.T., Bolton, E., Mays, V. and Goff, D. (2001). Cognitive therapy for psychosis in schizophrenia: an effect size analysis. *Schizophrenia Research, 48*, 335–342.

Haddock, G., McCarron, J., Tarrier, N. and Faragher, E.B. (1999). Scales to measure dimensions of hallucinations and delusions: the psychotic symptom rating scales (PSYRATS). *Psychological Medicine, 29*, 879–889.

Jones, G., Huckle, P. and Tanaghow, A. (1992). Command hallucinations, schizophrenia and sexual assaults. *Irish Journal of Psychological Medicine, 9*, 47–49.

Junginger, J. (1990). Predicting compliance with command hallucinations. *American Journal of Psychiatry, 147*, 245–247.

Kay, S.R., Fiszbein, A. and Opler, L.A. (1987). The positive and negative syndrome scale (PANSS) for schizophrenia. *Schizophrenia Bulletin, 13*, 261–269.

Kuipers, E., Fowler, D., Garety, P., Chisholm, D., Dunn, G., Bebbington, P., Freeman, D. and Hadley, C. (1998). The London–East Anglia randomised controlled trial of cognitive behaviour therapy for psychosis. III: Follow-up and economic evaluation at 18 months. *British Journal of Psychiatry, 173*, 61–68.

McGlashan, T.H. (1988). A selective review of North American long-term follow-up studies of schizophrenia. *Schizophrenia Bulletin, 14*, 515–542.

McGorry, P.D., Yung, A.R., Phillips, L.J. and Yuen, H.P. (2002). Randomised controlled trial of interventions designed to reduce the risk of progression to first episode psychosis in a clinical sample with sub-threshold symptoms. *Archives of General Psychiatry, 59*, 921–928.

Maden, A. (2003). Rethinking risk assessment. The MacArthur study of mental disorders and violence. *Psychiatric Bulletin, 27*, 237–238.

Milton, J., Amin, S., Sin, H.S., Harrison, G., Jones, P., Croudace, T., Medley, I. and Brewin, J. (2001). Aggressive incidents in first-episode psychosis. *British Journal of Psychiatry, 178*, 433–440.

Nelson, H.E. (1997). *Cognitive behaviour therapy with schizophrenia: a practice manual*. Cheltenham, UK: Stanley Thorne.

Norman, R. and Townsend, L. (1999). Cognitive-behavioural therapy for psychosis: a status report. *Canadian Journal of Psychiatry, 44*, 245–252.

Pilling, S., Bebbington, P., Kuipers, E., Garety, P., Beddes, J., Orbach, G. and Morgan, C. (2002). Psychological treatments in schizophrenia: I. Meta-analysis on family intervention and cognitive behavior therapy. *Psychological Medicine, 32*, 763–782.

Rooke, O. and Birchwood, M. (1998). Loss, humiliation and entrapment as appraisals of schizophrenic illness: a prospective study of depressed and non-depressed patients. *British Journal of Clinical Psychology, 37*, 259–268.

Rudnick-Abraham, S. (1999). Relation between command hallucinations and dangerous behaviour. *Journal of the American Academy of Psychiatry and Law, 27*, 253–257.

Sensky, T., Turkington, D., Kingdon, D., Scott, J.L., Siddle, R. and O'Carroll, M.

(2000). A randomised controlled trial of cognitive-behavioural therapy for persistent symptoms in schizophrenia resistant to medication. *Archives of General Psychiatry*, *57*, 165–172.

Shawyer, F., Mackinnon, A., Farhall, J., Trauer, T. and Copolov, D. (2003). Command hallucinations and violence: implications for detention and treatment. *Psychiatry, Psychology and Law*, *10*, 97–107.

Startup, M., Jackson, M. and Pearce, E. (2002). Assessing therapist adherence to cognitive-behaviour therapy for schizophrenia. *Behavioural and Cognitive Psychotherapy*, *30*, 329–339.

Tarrier, N., Kinney, C., McCarthy, E., Wittkowski, A., Yusopoff, L., Gledhill, A. and Morris, J. (2001). Are some types of psychotic symptoms more responsive to CBT? *Behavioural and Cognitive Psychotherapy*, *29*, 45–55.

Tarrier, N. and Wykes, T. (2004). Is there evidence that cognitive behaviour therapy is an effective treatment for schizophrenia? A cautious or cautionary tale? *Behaviour Research and Therapy*, *42*, 1377–1402.

Trower, P., Birchwood, M., Meaden, A., Byrne, S., Nelson, A. and Ross, K. (2004). Cognitive therapy for command hallucinations: randomized controlled trial. *British Journal of Psychiatry*, *184*, 312–320.

Trower, P. and Gilbert, P. (1989). New theoretical conceptions of social anxiety and social phobia. *Clinical Psychology Review*, *9*, 19–35.

Turkington, D., Kingdon, D. and Turner, T. (2002). Effectiveness of a brief cognitive-behavioural therapy intervention in the treatment of schizophrenia. *British Journal of Psychiatry*, *180*, 523–527.

Van der Gaag, M., Hageman, M.C. and Birchwood, M. (2003). Evidence for a cognitive model of auditory hallucinations. *Journal of Nervous and Mental Disease*, *191*, 542–545.

Appendix 1

Voice power differential scale (VPDS)
(Birchwood et al., 2000)

Client's Name: ....
Date Assessed: ....

Please circle the number which best describes how you feel in relation to your voice.
Name or description of voice: ....

1	2	3	4	5
I am much more powerful than my voice	I am more powerful than my voice	We have about the same amount of power as each other	My voice is more powerful than me	My voice is much more powerful than me
1	2	3	4	5
I am much stronger than my voice	I am stronger than my voice	We are as strong as each other	My voice is stronger than me	My voice is much stronger than me
1	2	3	4	5
I am much more confident than my voice	I am more confident than my voice	We are as confident as each other	My voice is more confident than me	My voice is much more confident than me
5	4	3	2	1
I respect my voice much more than it respects me	I respect my voice more than it respects me	We respect each other about the same	My voice respects me more than I respect it	My voice respects me much more than I respect it
1	2	3	4	5
I am much more able to harm my voice than it is able to harm me	I am more able to harm my voice than it is able to harm me	We are equally able to harm each other	My voice is more able to harm me than I am able to harm it	My voice is much more able to harm me than I am able to harm it
1	2	3	4	5
I am greatly superior to my voice	I am superior to my voice	We are equal to each other	My voice is superior to me	My voice is greatly superior to me

1	2	3	4	5
I am much more knowledgeable than my voice	I am more knowledgeable than my voice	We have about the same amount of knowledge as each other	My voice is more knowledgeable than me	My voice is much more knowledgeable than me

Appendix 2

Risk of Acting on Commands Scale (RACS) (Trower *et al.*, 2004)

Client's Name: ....

Date Assessed: ....

Low/No risk, low distress (Level 1)

Key criteria

1   No risk of acting on the command.
2   No distress associated with commands; PSYRATS rating of 1.

Evidence

1   Is able to fully resist commands.
2   Believes self to be more powerful than the voice/s, average Power Scale rating of 1 or 2.
3   Believes has a significant amount of control over the voice/s; rated as 80–100%.

Moderate risk, moderate distress (Level 2)

Key criteria

3   Moderate risk of acting on commands with potential harm to self or others: partial compliance/resistance to serious commands.
4   Low levels of distress associated with commands; PSYRATS rating of 1.

Evidence

4   Uses appeasement/coping strategies with potentially moderately serious consequences.
5   Believes self to be more powerful than the voice/s, average Power Scale rating of 2.
6   Believes has good control over the voice/s; rated as 60–80%.
7   Is able to resist voice commands on most occasions without fear of negative consequences.

Low risk, moderate distress (Level 3)

Key criteria

5   Low risk of acting on the command.
6   Moderate levels of distress associated with malevolent commands; PSYRATS rating of 2.

Evidence

8   May use subtle appeasement/coping strategies with less serious consequences.
9   Believes the voice to be more powerful that themselves in some respects but not in others OR to be equally powerful, average Power Scale rating of 3.
10 Believes has partial control over the voice/s; rated as 30–50%.
11 Is able to resist voice commands on most occasions but has some fear of negative (but not severe) consequences of resistance.

Moderate risk, moderate distress (Level 4)

Key criteria

7   Moderate risk of acting on the command with potential harm to self or others; partial compliance/resistance of serious commands.
8   Moderate levels of distress associated with malevolent commands; PSYRATS rating of 2.

Evidence

12 Uses appeasement/coping strategies with potentially moderately serious consequences.
13 Believes the voice to be more powerful than themselves in some respects but not in others OR to be equally powerful, average Power Scale rating of 3.
14 Believes has partial control over the voice/s; rated as 30–50%.
15 Believes that negative (but not severe) consequences will follow if the voice is not fully obeyed: the voice will inflict harm; resulting in partial compliance/ resistance.

Moderate risk, high distress (Level 5)

Key criteria

9   Moderate risk of acting on the command.
10 High levels of distress associated with malevolent commands; PSYRATS rating of 3 or 4.

Evidence

16 May use appeasement/coping strategies with less serious consequences; uses safety behaviours to neutralise the command or reduce anxiety in the short term.

17 Perceives the voice to be omnipotent and omniscient or very powerful; average Power Scale rating of 4 or 5.

18 Believes has little or no control over the voice; voice control rated as less than 20%.

19 Believes that the commands are morally repugnant and so should not be obeyed BUT fears severe consequences for non-compliance with commands.

High risk, high distress (Level 6)

Key criteria

11 High risk of acting on the command, with potential to harm self or others.

12 High levels of distress associated with malevolent commands; PSYRATS rating of 3 or 4.

Evidence

20 May use appeasement/coping strategies: resists more serious commands by enacting less serious behaviors (self-harm), or has the means to act on commands (carrying a knife).

21 Perceives the voice to be omnipotent and omniscient or very powerful; average Power Scale rating of 4 or 5.

22 Believes has little or no control over the voice; voice control rated as less than 20%.

23 Believes that severe consequences will follow if commands are not fully complied with; believes that the voice will inflict harm.

Appendix 3

CTCH – Therapy Adherence Protocol[1] (Trower et al., 2004)

Client: ....

Therapist: ....

Rater: ....

Date: ....

Rate all items on the following scale:

1	2	3	4	5
Not at all	Slightly	Moderately	Considerably	Extensively

Engagement phase

Establishment of rapport

Rating ☐

Did the therapist successfully establish rapport and trust: used empathic listening; explored beliefs and psychotic experiences in a non-judgemental way; helped the client feel understood?

Normalising

Rating ☐

Did the therapist help the client to recognise that their psychotic experiences are similar to the experiences of many people who have not been diagnosed with a mental illness?

Addressing engagement beliefs

Rating ☐

Did the therapist explore and address any beliefs that might threaten engagement: inability to change; resistance by voices; inability of the therapist to understand experiences?

---

1 Adapted from Startup, M., Jackson, M. and Pearce, E. (2002). Assessing therapist adherence to cognitive-behaviour therapy for schizophrenia. *Behavioural and Cognitive Psychotherapy*, *30*, 329–339.

Establishing the basis for intervention

Relocating the problem at B

Rating
☐

Did the therapist help the client to view the problem as a belief instead of hearing a voice *per se* and/or the emotional/behavioural distress associated with it?

Agreeing the beliefs to be targeted

Rating
☐

Did the therapist develop a collaborative description of the beliefs concerning power and compliance and agree which beliefs and in which order they would be tackled?

Clarifying the evidence for beliefs

Rating
☐

Did the therapist assess the evidence that the client uses to support the beliefs about power and compliance?

Intervention phase: Power, control and compliance beliefs

Reviewing and enhancing coping strategies

Rating
☐

Did the therapist systematically review the effectiveness of the client's coping strategies for addressing power imbalances, reducing compliance and improving control (i.e. reviewing when they were used, how consistently they were applied and how effective they were)? Were efforts subsequently made to improve these and introduce further strategies where appropriate?

Disputing power and compliance beliefs

Rating
☐

Did the therapist challenge the client's beliefs through discussion; offering challenges in a sensitive and tentative manner/'Columbo style'? Was there evidence that the therapist (a) highlighted logical inconsistencies in the belief system; (b) encouraged the client to consider alternative explanations?

Behavioural experiments/Reality testing

Rating
☐

Did the therapist encourage the client to seek disconfirmatory evidence and experiences? Did the therapist use RTHC? Was a clear behavioural experiment devised as a true test of the client's beliefs?

Advanced intervention I: Beliefs about identity, meaning/ purpose

Agreeing the beliefs to be targeted

Rating
☐

Did the therapist develop a collaborative description of the beliefs concerning Identity, Meaning/Purpose and agree which beliefs and in which order they would be tackled?

Clarifying the evidence for beliefs

Rating □

Did the therapist assess the evidence that the client uses to support the beliefs about Identity, Meaning and Purpose?

Disputing beliefs about identity, meaning/purpose

Rating □

Did the therapist challenge the client's beliefs through discussion; offering challenges in a sensitive and tentative manner/'Columbo style'? Was there evidence that the therapist (a) highlighted logical inconsistencies in the belief system; (b) encouraged the client to consider alternative explanations?

Behavioural experiments/Reality testing

Rating □

Did the therapist encourage the client to seek disconfirmatory evidence and experiences? Was a clear behavioural experiment devised as a true test of the client's beliefs?

Advanced intervention II: Self-evaluations

Exploring implications of psychotic beliefs for beliefs about self

Rating □

Did the therapist explore developmental and vulnerability factors that led to the development of psychotic experiences and beliefs?

Identifying core beliefs about self

Rating □

Did the therapist explore and identify the client's core self-beliefs: negative self-evaluations and dysfunctional assumptions? Did the therapist explore developmental and vulnerability factors that led to the development of core self-beliefs?

Connecting beliefs about identity, meaning/purpose to beliefs about self

Rating □

Did the therapist help the client to develop a personal model of his/her psychotic experiences based on a shared understanding of (a) the role of developmental and vulnerability factors in giving rise to and shaping core beliefs; (b) the role of psychotic experiences as a protective layer/defence?

Disputing core beliefs

Rating □

Did the therapist assess and dispute the evidence for the client's core beliefs; disputing the evidence; pointing out logical inconsistencies in the self-belief system; looking for alternative explanations? Did the therapist use specific philosophical disputation techniques: 'Big I little I'; evaluating behaviour vs whole-person evaluations; changing nature of self?

CTCH – Evaluation of treatment level attained

Tick each of the following treatment elements if they were completed during the course of therapy.

Engagement phase

Established rapport

☐

Successfully established rapport and trust: used empathic listening; explored beliefs and psychotic experiences in a non-judgemental way; helped the client feel understood?

Normalised

☐

Helped the client to recognise that their psychotic experiences were similar to the experiences of many people who have not been diagnosed with a mental illness?

Addressed engagement beliefs

☐

Explored and addressed any beliefs that threatened the engagement process: inability to change; resistance by voices; inability of the therapist to understand experiences?

Establishing the basis for intervention

Relocated the problem at B

☐

Helped the client to view the problem as a belief instead of hearing a voice *per se* and/or the emotional/behavioural distress associated with it?

Agreed the beliefs to be targeted

☐

Developed a collaborative description of the beliefs concerning power and compliance and agreed which beliefs and in which order they would be tackled?

Clarified the evidence for beliefs

☐

Assessed the evidence that the client used to support beliefs about power and compliance?

Intervention phase: Power, control and compliance beliefs

Reviewed and enhanced coping strategies

☐

Systematically reviewed the effectiveness of the client's coping strategies for addressing power imbalances, reduced compliance and improved control (i.e. reviewing when they were used; how consistently they were applied and how effective they were)? Improved coping strategies and introduced further strategies where appropriate?

Disputed power and compliance beliefs

Challenged beliefs through discussion; offered challenges in a sensitive and tentative manner/'Columbo style'? Highlighted logical inconsistencies in the belief system and encouraged the client to consider alternative explanations?

Behavioural experiments/Reality testing

Encouraged the client to seek disconfirmatory evidence and experiences? Used RTHC? Devised a behavioural experiment as a true test of the client's beliefs?

Advanced intervention I: Beliefs about identity, meaning/ purpose

Agreed the beliefs to be targeted

Developed a collaborative description of the beliefs concerning identity, meaning/ purpose and agreed which beliefs would be tackled and in which order?

Clarified the evidence for beliefs

Assessed the evidence that the client used to support beliefs about identity, meaning and purpose?

Disputed beliefs about identity, meaning/purpose

Challenged beliefs through discussion; offered challenges in a sensitive and tentative manner/'Columbo style'? Highlighted logical inconsistencies in the belief system and encouraged the client to consider alternative explanations?

Behavioural experiments/Reality testing

Encouraged the client to seek disconfirmatory evidence and experiences? Devised a behavioural experiment as a true test of the client's beliefs?

Advanced intervention II: Self-evaluations

Explored implications of psychotic beliefs for beliefs about self

Explored developmental and vulnerability factors that led to the development of psychotic experiences and beliefs?

Identified core beliefs about self

Explored and identified core self-beliefs: negative self-evaluations and dysfunctional assumptions? Explored developmental and vulnerability factors that led to the development of core self-beliefs?

Connected beliefs about identity, meaning/purpose to beliefs about self

Helped the client to develop a personal model of his/her psychotic experiences based on a shared understanding of (a) the role of developmental and vulnerability factors in giving rise to and shaping core beliefs; (b) the role of psychotic experiences as a protective layer/defence?

Disputed core beliefs

Assessed and disputed the evidence for the client's core beliefs; disputed the evidence; pointed out logical inconsistencies in the self-belief system; looked for alternative explanations? Used specific philosophical disputation techniques: 'Big I little I'; evaluating behaviour vs whole-person evaluations; changing nature of self?

Therapist: ....

Date: ....

Client: ....

No. of sessions: ....

CTCH – Individual session ratings

Client: ....

Therapist: ....

Rater: ....

Rate each session on all items (as applicable to the session) on the following scale:

1	2	3	4	5
Not at all	Slightly	Moderately	Considerably	Extensively

Engagement phase

Establishment of rapport

Sessions

1	2	3	4	5	6	7	8	9	10	11	12	13	14	15	16

Normalising

Sessions

1	2	3	4	5	6	7	8	9	10	11	12	13	14	15	16

Addressing engagement beliefs

Sessions

1	2	3	4	5	6	7	8	9	10	11	12	13	14	15	16

Establishing the basis for intervention

Relocating the problem at B

Sessions

1	2	3	4	5	6	7	8	9	10	11	12	13	14	15	16

Agreeing the beliefs to be targeted

Sessions

1	2	3	4	5	6	7	8	9	10	11	12	13	14	15	16

Clarifying the evidence for beliefs

Sessions

1	2	3	4	5	6	7	8	9	10	11	12	13	14	15	16

Intervention phase: Power, control and compliance beliefs

Reviewing and enhancing coping strategies

Sessions

1	2	3	4	5	6	7	8	9	10	11	12	13	14	15	16

Disputing power and compliance beliefs	Sessions															
	1	2	3	4	5	6	7	8	9	10	11	12	13	14	15	16

Behavioural experiments/Reality testing	Sessions															
	1	2	3	4	5	6	7	8	9	10	11	12	13	14	15	16

Advanced intervention I: Beliefs about identity, meaning/purpose

Agreeing the beliefs to be targeted	Sessions															
	1	2	3	4	5	6	7	8	9	10	11	12	13	14	15	16

Clarifying the evidence for beliefs	Sessions															
	1	2	3	4	5	6	7	8	9	10	11	12	13	14	15	16

Disputing identity/meaning/purpose beliefs	Sessions															
	1	2	3	4	5	6	7	8	9	10	11	12	13	14	15	16

Behavioural experiments/Reality testing	Sessions															
	1	2	3	4	5	6	7	8	9	10	11	12	13	14	15	16

Advanced intervention II: Self-evaluation

Exploring implications	Sessions															
	1	2	3	4	5	6	7	8	9	10	11	12	13	14	15	16

Identifying core self-beliefs	Sessions															
	1	2	3	4	5	6	7	8	9	10	11	12	13	14	15	16

Connecting psychotic beliefs to self	Sessions															
	1	2	3	4	5	6	7	8	9	10	11	12	13	14	15	16

Disputing core self-beliefs	Sessions															
	1	2	3	4	5	6	7	8	9	10	11	12	13	14	15	16

Index

abandonment 83
ABC model 11, 57, 79–80
abuse victims 27
abortion 50, 56, 71, 81–2
achievement 46, 67, 107
activity levels 58
activity scheduling 46
adolescence 60, 66; parental separation 66; stressful events 28; traumatic events 82; unwanted sexual incidents 95
affect 4
affection 71, 84; parental, lack of 82
aggression 8
agitation 56
agonic environment 8–9
alcohol 35; advantages and disadvantages of using 46; first experiments with 50; misused 39, 45
ambivalence 46, 52, 53
analogy 77, 85
anger 105; alleviating feelings of 106–7
anger management 106
animals 57
anxiety 11; acute 50, 99; alleviating feelings of 106–7; confronting 55, 58; coping with 27, 66; extreme 9, 56, 105; gradually subsided 44; reducing 23, 36, 52, 56, 80; severe symptoms 82; social 7; symptoms of 67, 75
anxiety management 75, 76, 102, 114; strategies 102; support 57, 59
appeasement 5, 7, 8, 9, 16, 26; reduced 21, 23, 34, 55; symbolic 17; strategies 22, 73
appraisals 6
arousal levels 106

assertiveness 28, 96, 107; recommendations for training 106
assessment 14, 21, 25–6, 31–2, 39–40, 50–2, 54, 60–2, 71–4, 89–91, 99–101; and formulation 7, 16–18
at risk register 70
attendance at therapy 52, 101; erratic 42, 48, 62
attention 76; craving 23; focusing away from voices 53; focusing on something of interest 42
atypicals 118
audio-tapes 18, 76
auditory hallucinations 1, 17–18, 50, 56; key beliefs about 17; severity of 29, 37, 48, 58, 68, 87, 97, 108
Australia 10
avoidant behaviours 45, 77

balanced lifestyle 56, 66, 108
BAVQ (*Beliefs about Voices Questionnaire*) 16–17, 112–13
Beck, A. T. 8, 10, 19
behavioural experiments 22
beliefs 4, 9, 11, 47; alternative 20, 43, 54; catastrophic 23; core 16; delusional 10; doubts about 21, 23, 30; dysfunctional 22, 23; facts and 15; functional 23; key 5, 7, 17; measured 17; questionable 24; religious 54; strengthening 23; targeted 30; testing 21, 23; weakening 23; *see also* compliance beliefs; control beliefs; identity beliefs; meaning beliefs; power beliefs; resistance beliefs
benevolence 5, 7, 9, 17, 82
bereavement 35, 56, 105
Birchwood, M. J. 4, 5, 7; *see also* BAVQ; CAS; OS; VPDS

Birmingham 112
blame 35, 72; punishment and 82
blaspheming 57
Bleuler, E. 1
BNF (British National Formulary)
    118
boredom: preventing 57, 67, 77
Braham, L. 4
brain 94, 104; erroneous activation of
    voice recognition centre 105;
    misinterpreting information 35, 45, 56,
    66, 82, 94; mistakes 57, 94; visual
    hallucinations triggered in 47; voices
    mistakenly generated by 108
breathing difficulty 75
breathing exercises 56, 66, 67, 76, 102,
    103
Brown, G. W. 7
bullies 25, 99, 104, 105, 106, 107, 108
Byrne, Sarah 31

cancer 27, 31, 104
cannabis 50
CAS (*Cognitive Assessment Schedule*) 17,
    112
catastrophe 22, 23
causal psychological mechanisms 11
CDSS (*Calgary Depression Scale for
    Schizophrenia*) 18, 72, 113
Chadwick, P. 4, 5, 10, 57; *see also* BAVQ;
    CAS
child abuse 24
childcare 70, 83–4
childhood 75; bullying 106; isolated 70;
    negative experiences 47; rape 19;
    stressful events 28; traumatic events 66
Clozapine 118
Cochrane plots 11
collaborative empiricism 10, 19
Columbo technique 21
commands: advantages and
    disadvantages of acting on 28, 44, 103,
    104; dangerous 11; definition of 14, 15;
    description of all 17; distressing 26;
    harmful 33, 65, 71, 74–5; harmless 17;
    high levels of distress associated with
    32; ignoring 23, 93; innocuous 6, 7, 17,
    61–2, 91; level of risk of acting on 18,
    32, 51, 73; minor 28; obeying 8, 42, 44,
    65, 96; perceived consequences of
    carrying out 23; questioning 23;
    resisting 22, 26, 40, 44, 65, 78, 80, 86,

93, 96, 103; selective sensitivity to 8;
    self-harm 25, 44, 68, 71, 101; serious
    22, 30, 70, 91; severe 2, 7, 17
commitment 15
compliance 1, 2, 5, 9, 16, 91; drug dose
    and 4; exploring beliefs around 28;
    greater likelihood of 6; level of 17;
    main behaviours targeted for
    intervention 26, 32, 40, 52, 62, 74, 91,
    101; partial 17, 73; perceived power
    differential that underpins the problem
    of 21; reducing 14, 21; risk of 6; voice
    will influence 4
compliance beliefs 19, 26, 32, 40, 42,
    51, 61–2, 73, 90, 100; exploring 28,
    33–4, 42–4, 53–5, 63–5, 78–81, 92–3,
    102–3
compulsion 14, 91, 99
concentration 76, 85; poor 86
concerns 52
confidentiality 96
confusion 56
continuing care 31
contradictory behaviour 21
contradictory messages 54
control 24, 34, 37, 48, 49, 68, 77, 85;
    exercise of 8; hearer does not have any
    16; promoting 14, 19–20, 23; regaining
    a sense of 14
control beliefs 19, 33, 41, 51, 61, 72, 90,
    100; challenging 26–7, 42, 53, 63, 76–7,
    91–2, 101–2; exploring 44, 65, 81, 93,
    103–4; significant positive change in
    69, 109
controllability 18
conviction 18, 21
coping 25, 35; difficulties in 60; loss of
    significant others 105; resources for 66;
    very limited ability 72; ways of 39, 42,
    46, 47, 60, 63, 76, 83, 91, 95
coping strategies 6, 20, 26, 34, 52, 81;
    costs and benefits of 46; different,
    exploring 41; enhancing 19; help
    reduce distress 44; help to identify 85;
    helpful 58; learning 27; range of 53;
    used more frequently 102; variety of
    67, 108; various 96
costs/benefits analysis 80
criminal content 2
crying 89, 105
cues 24
curiosity 21

danger 4, 34, 44
day centres 33, 42, 46, 48, 83, 88; referral
    to 77
death: father 31; fiancée/girlfriend 35;
    friends 50; grandfather 50, 104;
    grandmother 105; mother 27, 31, 35
delayed speech 75
delusions 17, 18; distress scale to compile
    total scores for 12; logical and
    empirical bases for 10; severity of 12,
    29, 37, 48, 58, 68, 87, 97, 108–9
dependent variables 11
depression 5, 11, 86; assessment of level
    of 18; easing 13; learning strategies for
    coping with 27; moderate 6, 39, 72;
    morning 18; observed 18, 72;
    postpsychotic 7; reduction in 12, 36;
    severe 39, 76; symptoms of 36, 76;
    theory developed to explain
    features of 7; trials measuring 12;
    understood in terms of vicious
    cycle 77
detention 2
diagnosis of schizophrenia 4, 18, 89, 94;
    ICD10 112
didactic techniques 19
disengagement option 15
disruption to life 18; severe 72
distraction techniques 33, 34, 42, 63,
    76–7, 101, 103, 107; useful 53
distress 6, 47, 49; alleviation of 12, 101;
    amount and intensity of 18, 37, 48, 58,
    87, 97, 109; changes over time 69;
    delusional 12; easing 13, 14;
    eradication of 11; high levels of 32, 40,
    51, 62, 73, 100; linked to voice activity
    5; more general measures for 17;
    perceived power differential that
    underpins the problem of 21; reducing
    11, 15, 19, 20, 21, 29, 41, 44, 62
disturbance 15; reducing 21
dominant voices 17, 50, 60, 71, 120;
    appeasing 116; male 89, 90, 99;
    powerful 100, 115, 116; response to
    91; severe commands from 113;
    wrath of 7
doubt 21, 23, 30, 37, 45, 55, 67
drug dose 4
Drury, V. 12
Dryden, W. 19
DSMIV (American Psychiatric
    Association) 1

dysfunctional behaviour 13; alleviation
    of 12; eradication or reduction of 11
dysfunctional schemas 8–9
dyslexia 70, 71, 76, 82

early wakening 18; severe 72
ECT (electroconvulsive therapy) 70, 76,
    85, 86
edgy feeling 75
education 56, 57, 66, 108; sex and social
    relationships 95, 106
elation 5
emotional dysfunction 13
empathic listening 15
empathy 82
enactment 22
encouragement 84
ending therapy 48
engagement 14, 15–16, 17, 18, 33, 40–1,
    52, 62, 74–6, 91, 101; help to cement
    20
entrapment 6
ethnic participants 113
evaluative themes 19
evidence 27; contradictory 21, 22;
    convincing 22, 43; questioning 22;
    resisting command voices 80
evolutionary psychology 7
expectations: concern about 15; family
    36; realistic 35
exploration 53, 57, 77, 85

family concerns 74–5
family contact 35, 36
fathers 35; absent 99, 105, 106;
    angry 99, 105; death of 31; good 92;
    irritable when tired 83; reprimand
    by 71
fear 5, 8, 26; exploration revealed 33
forensic services 2
formulation 14; assessment and 16–18;
    developing and sharing 18–19
frustration 106

genetic risk 94
gestures 17
Gilbert, P. 116
girlfriends 35, 50, 56
goals 11; questionable 10; research and
    practice 14; setting 14, 20
guided discovery 19, 21
guilt 5; pathological 18, 72

hallucinations *see* auditory hallucinations; olfactory hallucinations; tactile hallucinations; visual hallucinations
hallucinogenic drugs 56
hand-washing behaviour 99, 106–7
harm 2, 4, 14, 23, 28, 39, 54, 102; ability to 69; challenging beliefs about 78–9; commands to 30, 40, 42, 50, 52, 61, 65, 68, 71, 74–5, 101, 103; sexual 71; threats to 41, 42, 50; voice can inflict 16
hearers 6, 7, 19–20, 29; belief that voice is more powerful than 16; earplug use 53; perceived power of 24; talking about their experiences 41; voice can inflict harm on 16
helplessness 84
homework tasks 33, 42, 101
homosexuality 106
hopelessness 18, 72
hospitalisation 2, 4, 50, 60, 76, 99, 113–14; sometimes necessary 72
hot flushes 75
household chores 70–1
hypotheses 21, 82

ICD10 diagnosis 112
idealisation 23
ideas of reference 18
identity 5–6, 7, 21, 30; attributed to school bullies 106; doubts about 37, 55
identity beliefs 16, 17, 19, 24, 26, 32, 40, 51, 62, 73, 86, 90–1, 100–1; exploring 28, 35–6, 45, 56–7, 66–7, 82, 94–5; significant changes in 108
illegal drugs 50, 56
inconsistencies 21, 22
independence 95, 104
inferences 21, 23
inferiority 9
inherited mental mechanisms 8
inner speech 82; misattributed 35, 45, 56, 66, 82, 94; voices might reflect 66
interpretations 21
intervention 1, 7, 16, 21–5, 26–30, 31, 33–6, 37, 40–5, 52–7, 62–7, 74–82, 91–5, 101–5; assessment and 20; evaluating the outcome of 14; gauging the impact of 18; guiding 2, 11; main compliance behaviours targeted for 26, 32, 40, 52, 62, 74, 91, 101

irritability 75, 83
isolation 82

Jones, G. 4
Junginger, J. 6

killing 2, 25, 27, 28, 50, 51, 52, 53–4, 61; attempted 114

learning difficulties 70, 82, 98; moderate 89; problems at school due to 66
learning strategies 27
logical reasoning 22
loneliness 67, 82
loss 12, 83; coping with 105
loud voices 43, 51, 64, 93; aggressive 34, 41, 54, 102; distressing 60; extreme 39, 50, 60; frequent 8, 27, 73, 107; nasty 96; negative 99; persistent 8, 25, 44; unpleasant 89, 99
Lowe, C. F. 10

MacArthur study 4
McGorry, P. D. 12
malevolence 5, 7, 9, 17, 30, 81
marriage difficulty 39
mastery 24
meaning 6, 7; constructed by individuals 5; purpose and 16
meaning beliefs 17, 19, 26, 32, 37, 40, 51, 62, 74, 91, 100–1; exploring 28, 35, 45, 55–6, 66, 81–2, 94, 105; significant changes in 108
medication 31, 33, 56; combined with relaxation 85; monitoring 76; new 83, 86; proxy drug that can be conveniently compared to 11; taken regularly 42, 66, 77, 95; very high dose 4
memory problems/difficulties 76, 85
Mental Health Act (1983) 113–14
mental states 17, 18
mentalities 8
messengers from God 51, 53, 56
meta-analyses 11
mind reading 47
mood 79; depressed 18, 36, 37, 46, 67, 80, 81; improvement in 12; low 45, 57, 77
motivation 16
multiple baseline single-case methodology 10
music: relaxing 34, 52, 91, 101; useful distraction technique 53

negative events 36, 57
Nelson, Angela 112, 113
Nelson, H. E. 35, 43, 45, 53, 56, 57, 66, 79, 82, 94, 104
neuroleptics 11–12
non-compliance 22
non-forensic patients 2
novel ideas 19
nurturing 82

obedience 7; likely consequences of 17
OCD (obsessive-compulsive disorder) 99
olfactory hallucinations 67
omnipotence 5, 16; beliefs around 23, 24; challenging 14; perceived 6, 9
omniscience 7; beliefs around 23
OS (*Omniscience Scale*) 17
outcome 14, 28–30, 31, 36–7, 58–9, 68–9, 85–7, 96–7, 108–9; feared 23
overdoses 26, 50, 54

panic alarms 42
panic attacks 75
PANSS (*Positive and Negative Syndrome Scale*) 17, 111, 113, 117, 118
paranoia 50, 52; confronting 55
past relationships 47
persecution 9; for past misdemeanours 28
personification 7, 9, 14, 23
pharmacological studies 11
physical sensations 67
Pilling, S. 12
positive achievements 36
post-traumatic memories 105
power 5, 9, 19, 27; components of 17; control and 16; exercise of 8; interpersonal appraisal of 6; perceived 6, 21, 24; promotion of 23; proof of 7
power beliefs 17, 18, 20, 21, 23, 24, 32, 39, 51, 61, 72, 90, 100; exploring 34, 44, 55, 65, 81, 93, 103–4; overall 48; significant positive changes in 109
powerlessness 6, 20, 28, 33, 48, 54, 55, 65, 79, 81, 102
PQRST (*Personal Questionnaire Rating Scale Technique*) 12
prediction 7, 22, 61
predisposition 35, 45, 56, 66, 82, 94, 105
preoccupation 18
preparatory acts 17

problem-solving 36, 46, 56, 57, 77, 102; worrying and 107–8
psychosis 4, 9; easing distress and depression in 13; eradication or amelioration of symptoms of 11; one of the most intractable problems in 10; secondary appraisals of 12
PSYRATS (*Psychotic Symptom Rating Scales*) 12, 17–18, 28, 29, 37, 48, 58, 68, 87, 97, 108, 113, 116
punishment 6, 7, 21, 26, 35, 37, 40, 81; blame and 82; deserved 19; fear of 19, 22; ignoring commands without 24; past behaviour 16, 66; severe 23; threat of 8
purpose 17; beliefs about 19, 26

quality time 84
quasineuroleptic approach 10–13

RACS (*Risk of Acting on Commands Scale*) 18
radio 53
randomised controlled trials 10, 18, 111–19
rape 60; childhood 19; self-blame for 82; traumatic, psychological reaction to 24; violent 71
rapport 15
rational emotive behaviour therapy 4, 19
reality testing 22
redundancy 35
reformulation 24; tentative 19
relationship difficulties 45
relaxation exercises 56, 63, 66, 76, 102, 103; medication combined with 85
relief 73; immediate 20
reprimand 71
resistance 9, 16, 28; easing distress associated with 14; emphasising benefits of 23; increased 21; level of 17; likely consequences of 17
resistance beliefs 26, 32, 40, 51, 61–2, 73, 90, 100; exploring 33–4, 42–4, 53–5, 63–5, 78–81, 92–3, 102–3
ridicule 47
RMOs (responsible medical officers) 118
Rooke, O. 7
rumination 57

safety behaviours 5, 7, 22, 23
safety precautions 41, 42

Sandwell 112
schizophrenia 95; CBT an established therapy for 10; diagnosis of 4, 18, 89, 94, 112
secret friends 71
self-blame 82, 105
self-concept 25
self-confidence 69, 98; low 66, 67
self-depreciation 18, 72; severe 72
self-harm 2, 7, 34, 85; commands to 25, 44, 68, 71; denied 51; likely 32, 62, 73; risk of 4
self-talk technique 67
semi-secure units 2, 112
sensitivity 104
sexual abuse/assault 9, 25, 26, 66, 67, 81, 89, 94
sexual intercourse 95
sexual orientation 106
shaking 75
shame 12
Shawyer, F. 1, 2
silence 53
sleep 77, 108; better 37; difficulties 107; preparation 34; voices worse when trying to 67
sociability 58
Social Comparison Scale 8
social rank theory 7, 16; agonic dominant/subordinate perspective 8
social services 70, 83
social status 6
social transgressions 6; major 7; minor 2
socialisation to the cognitive model 15–16, 18
Socratic questioning/dialogue 19, 24, 33, 43, 53, 64, 65, 78, 94, 103, 104; powerful form of 21
Solihull 112
special needs 71, 99, 108
stimulants 56, 66; avoiding 92, 95
stimulation 86
stress: build-up of 105, 108; coping with 35, 37, 56, 66, 85; events in childhood and adolescence 28; extreme, response to 35; resources for coping with 108; visual hallucinations triggered in brain by 47
stress management 35, 56, 66
stress/vulnerability model 35, 45, 66, 82, 94, 105

submission 8
subordination 5, 6, 8
suicide 11; attempted, elevated risk of 18; deliberately considered 72
superiority 69, 90, 100, 109
supernatural force 5
support 28, 48–9, 89, 105; community mental health services 50; day and night access to 26
support networks 35; encouragement to extend 83; good, maintaining 46, 56, 66, 85, 108
symptoms 1, 4; alleviation of 12; amount and intensity of distress associated with 29, 37, 48, 58, 87, 97, 109; assessment of 14; decisive impact on 12; disclosing information about 15; more general measures for 17; negative 18; positive 12, 13; predisposition to 35, 56; reduction or removal of 12; trials traditionally aimed at reducing 11
systemic work 84–5

tactile hallucinations 56, 67
target behaviours 26, 32, 40, 52, 62, 74, 91, 101
Tarrier, N. 12
TAU (treatment as usual) 112, 114, 115, 116, 118
Ten Commandments 54
therapeutic alliance/relationship 15, 20, 76
Therapy Adherence Protocol 18
thoughts 7; anxious 75; automatic 35, 45, 46, 56, 66, 82, 94; blaspheming 57; intrusive 57; negative 45, 66, 77, 82; previously unspoken 35
threats 54; de-escalating 8; empty 43, 79; personal 25
trauma 19, 35, 66; rape 24
traumatic memories 67
treatment resistant people 2
trials 11, 12, 31, 85; randomised 10, 18, 111–19
triggers 24, 28, 36, 37, 45, 46, 47, 57, 67, 82, 83, 94, 95, 106; bereavement 35; drug use 66; external sound 53, 58; higher or lower numbers of stressful events 56; panic 75
Trower, P. E. 4, 7, 10

trust 28, 36, 41, 46; abuse of 19;
    establishing 15
TV watching 53

understanding 91; shared 19, 21, 132,
    135
unpleasant past events 104
upbringing of children 39, 84, 99; less
    than ideal 83

validity testing 22
Van der Gaag, M. 5
VCS (*Voice Compliance Scale*) 17, 113
verbal abuse 25
verbalisation 77
vicious circles 36
vicious cycle 45, 77
video-taping 18
violence 60, 66; increased risk of 2
visual hallucinations 50, 56; triggered 47,
    57
voice content 4, 5, 46; client's
    interpretation of 19; discussed 44;
    doubting the truth of 64, 92; inability
    to control 58; negative 60–1, 72, 83, 89,
    99–100; unpleasant 60–1, 72, 89,
    99–100
voices: absence of 83; aggressive 34, 41;
    almost continuous 39, 50, 60, 72;
    appraisal of 5; assertiveness with 28;
    challenging the reliability of 79;
    command(ing) 1, 2, 15, 16, 17, 28,
    33–4, 85; convincingly real 67; critical
    61, 72; depressed mood and 45–6;
    dimensions of relationship with 17;
    direct challenge to 43; distressing 24,

66, 68, 72, 82, 85, 86, 89, 105, 108; first
    hearing 31, 39, 50, 60, 89; frequent 8,
    25, 27, 42, 71, 72, 73, 108; frightening
    60, 72, 90; helpful and comforting 71,
    82; learning to start and stop at will 19;
    nasty 71, 82; normalising 22, 23;
    obeying 16, 44; overdoses in response
    to 26; persistent 8, 25, 27, 40, 43, 44;
    quietening 77; remission from 25, 31;
    respected 39, 72, 100; risks associated
    with talking about 41; screaming 73;
    shadowing 42, 102; shouting 50, 60,
    73, 74; significant others and 9, 28;
    silent 79; swearing 50, 71; switching on
    and off 23–4, 53; temporarily silencing
    73; threat posed by 7, 58, 63, 85;
    unpleasant 71, 87; *see also*
    appeasement; beliefs; benevolence;
    commands; compliance; control;
    dominant voices; hearers; loud voices;
    malevolence; omnipotence;
    persecution; personification; power
VPDS (*Voice Power Differential Scale*)
    17, 25, 28–9, 32, 37, 39, 48, 51, 58, 61,
    68, 72, 87, 90, 97, 100, 108, 113
vulnerability 94; cognitive 9; potential 95

warmth 82
West Midlands 112
withholding behaviour 22
working in excess 35
worrying 107–8
worthlessness 19, 72
wrist-cutting 26, 61, 73, 86, 100

youth custody 25